# The Weight's Over, Take Back Control

# The Weight's Over, Take Back Control

## Ditch dieting, transform your mindset and change your life

Sandra Roycroft-Davis

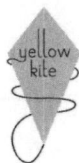

yellow kite

First published in Great Britain in 2025 by Yellow Kite
An imprint of Hodder & Stoughton Limited
An Hachette UK company
The authorised representative in the EEA is Hachette Ireland, 8 Castlecourt
Centre, Dublin 15, D15 XTP3, Ireland (email: info@hbgi.ie)

1

A CIP catalogue record for this title is available from the British Library

Trade Paperback ISBN 9781399731133
ebook ISBN 9781399731140

Typeset in Celeste by Hewer Text UK Ltd, Edinburgh
Printed and bound in Great Britain by Clays Ltd, Elcograf S.p.A.

Hodder & Stoughton policy is to use papers that are natural, renewable
and recyclable products and made from wood grown in sustainable
forests. The logging and manufacturing processes are expected to
conform to the environmental regulations of the country of origin.

Hodder & Stoughton Limited
Carmelite House
50 Victoria Embankment
London EC4Y 0DZ

www.yellowkitebooks.co.uk

# Contents

## PART ONE: WHAT DIETING DOES TO YOU

**CHAPTER 1:**

**CHAPTER 2:**

**CHAPTER 3:**

**CHAPTER 4:**

**CHAPTER 5:**

**CHAPTER 6:**

# CONTENTS

# Foreword

As a clinician working in the NHS in a hospital setting and as someone who has many patients with weight-related challenges, it is a privilege to work with Sandra, whose programme has benefited more than 350,000 people.

Sandra has nearly two decades of experience and success in helping people to implement strategies that enable them to achieve a healthier lifestyle and weight. The lessons she shares in this book, which are potentially transformational, will help anyone who is struggling with their weight or stuck in the endless cycle of yo-yo dieting, as well as healthcare professionals and clinicians across the world.

This book is most definitely a game changer, with a focus on the experience of people who struggle to achieve and maintain a healthy weight, and introducing tools that actually work and are accessible to everyone. I would recommend that you take a look . . .

Professor Adrian Heald
Consultant Endocrinologist, Salford Royal Hospital
Visiting Tutor, St Peters College, Oxford

# A Bit About Me

Hi, I'm Sandra.

I am the creator of the clinically proven, medically endorsed Slimpod programme, which has over 350,000 users. The success of the programme won me the award of Best Businesswoman in Health & Beauty in 2024. I'm an NHS collaborator and a leading Harley Street behavioural change specialist, with almost two decades of experience in transforming the lives of people who are exhausted with dieting and want to discover a better way to lose weight naturally and sustainably. I am a sought-after speaker for international health conferences in London, Dubai, Milan and Prague and have appeared on *ITV Tonight* and Channel 4's *How to Lose Weight Well*. In this book, I will share my wealth of experience to empower you to shift your mindset, gain a healthier attitude towards food and finally lose weight for good.

*Sandra*
x

# Introduction

I'm sitting in my therapy room in Harley Street on a rainy day in September 2009. I'm with a lady who's been dieting for more than 30 years and is really struggling with her mental health. She tells me she's put on the same three stone over and over again, and is now the heaviest she's ever been.

This lady has become obsessed with food, is addicted to weighing herself daily and is constantly self-sabotaging because she's now become a comfort eater. She feels a failure, her self-esteem is at rock bottom and she tells me she's given up believing she can ever lose weight.

Sadly, this is such a familiar story. So many people I see for one-to-one therapy have the same problem with their mental health because years of dieting have psychologically damaged their relationship with food. I resonate completely with them because, when I was younger, I was in the same position and my self-esteem also suffered.

## From Struggle Comes Hope

I was an overweight child and I'll never forget the way I was bullied at school because of my size. They called me 'Miss Piggy' in the playground and that stuck with me for many, many years.

Chocolate became more than a treat for me. It was my comfort, my escape, leading me into a downward spiral of guilt and further indulgence. It was tough. I struggled with rock-bottom confidence and my low self-esteem stayed with me way into adult life. I used to tell myself I was useless, worthless, that nobody liked me – I felt I had no friends. This would drive me into a vicious circle where I'd eat even more chocolate and become even more miserable.

Yet, through my own painful battles, I equipped myself with the tools of behavioural change, transforming my inner struggle into a beacon of hope for others. The most important lesson I learned is that sustainable weight loss is about so much more than how much – or what – you put on your plate.

The brain plays a huge part in your success – you need to know how to retrain it to think differently about the lifestyle you desire.

In Harley Street, I helped my patients understand what is holding them back and how we need to get their mind and body working together again, instead of fighting each other, so they start losing weight in a sustainable way.

It was with this knowledge that I developed the Slimpod programme in 2010, a culmination of personal growth and professional expertise, to help more people to take back control of their lives. To date, more than 350,000 people have been on the programme and, for many, it's been a life-changing process.

## Why We All Need To Do Something

Since the 1960s, consumers have spent billions trying to lose weight and yet, in the UK alone, latest government figures show that *three-quarters* of people over the age of 40 are overweight or obese.[1] Many of them will have spent 25 years or more on a diet of some kind.

Worldwide, more than *two billion* people are overweight and over 600 million of those are obese.[2] In the United States, more than 100 million people are on a diet and, in the UK, 55 per cent of the adult population is on a diet at any one time. The average dieter spends over £30,000 on diets in their lifetime and yet these are the people who are most likely to be overweight later in life.[3] Obesity has now become a bigger problem than malnutrition, and type 2 diabetes is at an all-time high. Some 96 per cent of people with diabetes are over 40.[4]

One of the scariest stats of all is this: among the obese people who try to lose weight, the failure rate is 99 per cent.[5] And, sadly, for the other 1 per cent, the success is only temporary. The vast majority of dieters end up heavier than when they started.[6]

If this happened in any other walk of life there would be outrage. If a school, college or university had a 99 per cent failure rate it would be closed down – the same with a hospital or business. There's a huge disconnect.

Millions of people are clearly motivated to lose weight.

Many of them are so desperate that it causes mental health issues. But when they get into their forties they're exhausted. They feel out of control because they've tried everything and find themselves bigger than they were when they started dieting decades earlier.

Over the years, their positive body image has been eroded away because food has become the enemy and the body the battleground. They're desperate and they feel helpless. They've stopped believing life can be any different and they now believe they'll be fat for the rest of their lives. They've been disempowered and have stopped trusting themselves around food. They have no idea what it's like to be a 'normal' eater anymore. Sadly, most people's relationship with food is now based on emotion rather than logic.

Clearly, something is stopping the over-forties from losing weight, from being healthier and happier. And the reason is a mystery for so many people. They are hypnotised by diets and the food industry, and have no idea how to break free from the trance and get their lives back. If this resonates with you, read on as that's what this life-changing book is about: freedom, liberation and, above all, hope.

## The Weight's Over

Recently, I asked some of our Slimpod members to complete a survey I called the 'Diet Dossier'. Nearly 4,000 responded and it revealed incredible information about the effects of dieting and their relationship with food – and themselves – before they came on to my programme. Their deeply personal insights into what dieting has done to them convinced me to write this book, to help more people realise that constantly having their weight on their minds is what prevents them from achieving sustainable weight loss. I firmly believe this is one of the reasons for the current obesity epidemic.

People have been conditioned to think that, if they follow this diet or that one, take this pill or that one, or have this jab or that one, then they'll magically lose weight. Well, yes, many do get instant weight loss. But for 95 per cent of them it doesn't last.[7] Day-to-day life, stress, anxiety and boredom lead to emotional eating and they go back to square one, feeling like a failure again. It's a horrible cycle that takes a heavy toll on their well-being.

This book is a testament to the power of positivity. It's a guide that aims not only to inform, but to inspire. Everything you'll discover in the book is based on scientific research and, throughout these pages, we'll delve into the innermost parts of our minds, unravelling the tangled threads of thoughts and feelings that shape our self-perception. How we see ourselves is the key to contentment. Once we can throw off the shackles of how we think others see us, a new perspective on life opens up. What's between our ears is the missing piece of the weight-loss puzzle. Our brains can block weight loss or they can be our greatest asset.

To retrain your brain to have a better relationship with food you need to take a leap of faith and be open-minded to learn more, ready to have your life changed. Many people have done just that and you'll see their stories running through the book because they're a constant inspiration to me and many others – I'm so very proud of them and what they're achieving. I love celebrating their success because they've been there, done it and got the smaller T-shirt. They are what drives me on my mission to help people understand there is a happier way to live their lives rather than going mindlessly from one meal to the next and panicking about everything that passes their lips.

Life really doesn't have to be that way at all.

When you understand how you can change yourself, it's so empowering. You'll be part of your own journey to health and you'll become a huge part of the solution. You then have choices and optimism about the future. It's like walking through the wardrobe door and into Narnia – a whole new world opens up and it changes everything.

You may have read weight-loss books before. You've probably tried a diet or two without success. If you've given up on losing weight, read on – this book is different and it's all about giving you hope and showing you that you *can* take back control.

I've split the book into three parts. First, we look at the most common issues faced by people trying to lose weight. Then, we discover why the way you are really isn't your fault. Finally, you'll be ready for my magic sauce: the proven ways you can take control of your eating and your life. All the way through you'll find expert tips to guide you.

So, let's walk through the wardrobe door together because, finally, the weight's over. This is the moment you start to take back control.

# PART ONE

# What Dieting Does to You

These first chapters unravel the top negative psychological effects of dieting based on my experience over nearly two decades and the responses to my Diet Dossier survey. I'll be explaining where it's all gone so wrong and how to change things. I'll show that you *can* reverse this and take back control!

Let's begin by looking at the issue dieters rank as their number one problem, one which keeps them going round and round in circles for years: self-sabotage.

CHAPTER 1

# Why 85 Per Cent of People Self-Sabotage

Why is it that just when you start to see progress on your weight-loss journey, you suddenly find yourself sabotaging your own efforts? I've witnessed this so often over the years and, in my Diet Dossier survey, self-sabotage was the top reason, given by 85 per cent of people, for why they couldn't sustain diets. However, I know that understanding the psychological and emotional dynamics at play can help them – and now you – navigate through and beyond self-sabotage.

## What is Self-Sabotage?

Self-sabotage is not just about a lack of willpower or knowledge; it's deeply rooted in psychological and emotional responses to dieting.[1] Whether it's skipping a planned workout or binge eating, these behaviours often stem from an inner resistance to change, fear of the unknown or comfort in familiarity, even when it's detrimental.

There are three major psychological underpinnings for self-sabotage:

## Fear of change

Contrary to popular belief, the fear of success can be as daunting as the fear of failure. Achieving weight-loss goals often brings about significant life changes, including new self-expectations, shifts in relationships and altered identities.

These changes can feel overwhelming, leading to a subconscious retreat to old habits to avoid confronting new challenges. Research indicates that emotional responses to weight change can trigger behaviours that hinder weight-loss goals.[2]

## Unrealistic goals

Setting overly ambitious goals is a common pitfall. Unrealistic expectations can lead to frustration and decreased motivation when results aren't immediate or dramatic. This cycle often culminates in the abandonment of weight-loss efforts.

Studies have shown that those with unrealistic weight-loss expectations are more likely to drop out of weight-loss programmes, often following periods of negative self-evaluation and compensatory behaviours like binge eating.[3]

## Lack of coping mechanisms

Stress is a well-documented trigger for behaviours that counteract weight-loss efforts.[4] Without effective coping strategies, you may turn to food for comfort, using it as a mechanism to manage negative emotions.

Emotional eating undermines diet and health goals, acting as a significant form of self-sabotage. Understanding and accepting that setbacks are a natural part of the journey to a healthier lifestyle is essential.

Learning from setbacks, rather than using them as an excuse to revert to old habits, is key. Each lapse provides valuable insights into vulnerabilities and how to manage them more effectively in the future.

Not only that, being kind to yourself can ease the process. Self-compassion encourages you to forgive yourself for setbacks and view them as opportunities for growth and learning, rather than reasons for self-criticism and defeat.

Self-sabotage is a multi-faceted issue influenced by psychological, emotional and habitual factors. What I am sharing in this book will help you to address these root causes, because with realistic goal-setting, healthy stress-management techniques and enhanced self-awareness, you can better navigate your weight-loss journey and achieve lasting health improvements.

Recognising and understanding the patterns of self-sabotage are the first steps towards developing a healthier relationship with food and oneself. Embrace the strategies below with a positive mindset, and watch as you transform your relationship with food and achieve your weight-loss goals.

Believe in your ability to make lasting changes and take it one step at a time. You've got this!

### How You Can Take Back Control
*Set realistic and achievable goals*
One of the most effective strategies to prevent self-sabotage is setting goals that are both realistic and sustainable. Goals should adhere to the SMART criteria: Specific,

Measurable, Attainable, Relevant and Time-bound. We'll discuss goal-setting in more detail in Chapter 24. Celebrating small victories can also provide motivation and positive reinforcement, helping to maintain momentum.

### Develop healthy ways to cope

Since stress can trigger self-sabotaging behaviour, developing healthy coping mechanisms is crucial. Techniques such as mindfulness, deep breathing exercises and yoga can alleviate stress without resorting to food. Cognitive behavioural therapy (CBT) is also beneficial for altering thought patterns that lead to self-sabotage.

### Enhance self-awareness

Keeping a detailed food and mood diary can help identify triggers for self-sabotaging behaviours. A trigger could be the smell of fresh bread, the sight of a cream cake, the sound of bacon sizzling or even a parent's voice awakening childhood memories of chocolate. Keeping a diary increases self-awareness and helps individuals understand the link between their emotions and eating habits. Recognising these patterns is the first step towards changing them.

### Build a support system

Involving a support system can encourage positive behaviour and provide accountability. Friends, family or professional counsellors can offer support and feedback crucial for overcoming moments of weakness.

## Case Study: How I Took Back Control

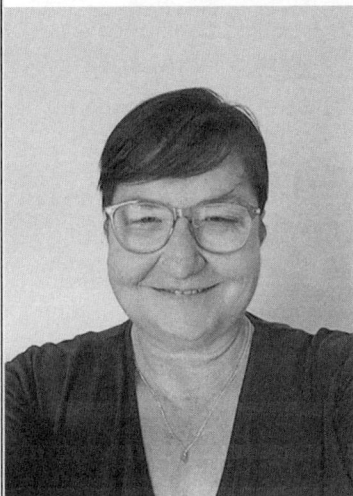

*Jane Foster*

I had hit rock bottom. I would sit in the car park of the local shop, hiding in plain sight, and devour an entire Victoria sponge cake with my hands. It was a secret, desperate act. I felt completely unworthy, like a failure, and food became my way of punishing myself.

I was trapped in a cycle of self-destruction, too exhausted and overwhelmed to even consider a way out. My life was ruled by unhealthy habits – bingeing on processed food, drinking too much and dressing in a way that mirrored how I felt inside: defeated and uncaring.

My days blurred together as I chose quick, convenient meals, just to avoid the effort of preparing something myself.

I was always tired, always aching and constantly struggling with health issues that landed me in and out of hospital. I was stuck in this awful loop, feeling powerless and resigned to a future of deteriorating health.

But then, something shifted. I can't say exactly when it happened, but I realised that I was tired of being tired. I began tapering off my medication, even though it was hard, and I pushed myself to cook a meal every day. It wasn't easy, but I discovered that I wasn't as helpless as I'd thought. Slowly, I started taking back control, proving to myself that I could change my life, one small step at a time.

This wasn't about losing weight or fitting into a smaller dress size – although that did happen. I went from a size 24 down to a size 16 and, I won't lie, it felt good. But the real victory was regaining my health and, more importantly, my confidence. I stopped needing painkillers, my blood sugar levels normalised and my blood pressure stabilised. I was able to come off several medications, including those for diabetes and high cholesterol. My doctors were amazed at the transformation, but, to me, the most significant change was that I no longer felt like a passenger in my own life.

Today, I approach life with a sense of purpose and determination. I've learned that consistency is key – not just in eating healthier but in the mindset I bring to each day. My goal isn't to be slim; it's to be healthy, to be strong and to never go back to that dark place where I had given up on myself.

*Find out more about Jane's story here:*

## CHAPTER 2

# Don't Let the Scales Dictate Your Mood

Many of us have experienced the cycle of anxiety that comes with daily weigh-ins. You step on the scales, hoping to see progress, and your mood for the day hinges on the number displayed. I certainly witness this every day within our Slimpod community. And over time it becomes addictive.

So why do we become so fixated on a figure? Why does it become an addiction for so many people and one of the main reasons for self-sabotage?

In the Diet Dossier, obsessing over scale weight was the second most common negative effect of dieting, with 3,100 people (82 per cent) saying they did this. Of these, 37 per cent said they weighed once a day, 29 per cent said once a week and 23 per cent said two or three times a week.

## The Brain's Reward System

When you last began a diet, did you become preoccupied with the scales? This common fixation is not merely a trivial habit; it's rooted in complex brain functions. Sustainable weight loss, however, is not about restricting what you eat and then obsessing about the number on the scales. It's about improving your overall well-being and forming lasting, healthy habits. By understanding more about the impact of dieting and weighing on your brain, it can help you reclaim control and foster a healthier relationship with food and weight loss.

To truly understand the power the scales have over you, we need to delve into the psychological and neurological processes that come into play. The brain's reward system plays a significant role in this obsession. Each time you see a lower number on the scale, your brain releases dopamine, the 'feel-good' neurotransmitter associated with pleasure and reward. This dopamine release reinforces the behaviour, creating a reward loop. This reinforcement can make daily weigh-ins a habit, as you seek that dopamine hit from seeing progress.

Dieting also primes your brain to focus on specific outcomes, like weight loss. This priming makes you more attentive to the scales, looking for confirmation that your efforts are paying off. This confirmation bias makes you overly sensitive to small weight fluctuations, interpreting them as significant successes or failures. Cognitive biases can significantly influence perception and decision-making, leading to an unhealthy preoccupation with weight.[1]

The emotional rollercoaster linked to the scales can be intense. Seeing a decrease in weight can elate you, while an increase can bring disappointment or frustration. These emotional highs and lows can make you dependent on the scales for validation, impacting your mood and self-esteem. This emotional dependency can derail your long-term goals by causing stress and anxiety, which are counterproductive to sustainable weight loss.

By understanding the brain's role in weight loss, you can transform your relationship with the scales. Sustainable weight loss is about more than just the numbers. It's about fostering a healthier mindset and embracing a balanced approach to well-being.

It's essential to shift your focus from the scales to other indicators of progress. Redirect your attention to non-scale victories, such as increased energy levels, improved fitness, better sleep and how your clothes fit. Celebrating these wins reinforces positive behaviours without relying solely on weight. Keeping a record of these wins can help you stay motivated and recognise the many benefits of your efforts.

Another practical strategy is to limit your weigh-ins. Instead of daily weigh-ins, try reducing the frequency to once a week or even less. This approach minimises the impact of minor daily fluctuations and helps you focus on long-term trends. Research suggests that less frequent weigh-ins can reduce anxiety and promote a healthier perspective on weight loss.[2]

My advice is to ditch the scales if you have an unhelpful emotional reaction to them. Hide them in a cupboard so that your mood can no longer be dictated by a lump of plastic, metal or glass lurking in the bathroom.

## How You Can Take Back Control

*Shift your focus to other wins*

Celebrate non-scale wins like increased energy, better sleep, improved fitness and how your clothes fit. Keeping a journal of these wins can help you recognise the many benefits of your efforts and keep you motivated.

*Limit your weigh-ins*

Reduce the frequency of your weigh-ins to once a week or less. This approach helps you focus on long-term trends rather than daily fluctuations, reducing anxiety and promoting a healthier perspective on weight loss.

*Set holistic goals*

Broaden your goals beyond weight loss to include overall health and well-being. Focus on developing healthy habits like regular exercise, balanced nutrition and adequate sleep. Setting holistic goals helps maintain perspective and prioritise long-term health over short-term weight changes.

*Use cue-routine-reward*

Modify the habit loop that leads you to weigh yourself daily. Identify the cue, change the routine to something positive like mindful meditation or stretching, and establish a new reward. Maybe every morning and evening, when you brush your teeth, you see the bathroom scales. Lock them out of sight! Don't record weight lost in your diary of daily wins; record clothes becoming looser instead, so that how you feel becomes the habit, not how much you weigh. This approach can disrupt the habit of daily weigh-ins and build a healthier, more supportive routine.

## Case Study: How I Took Back Control

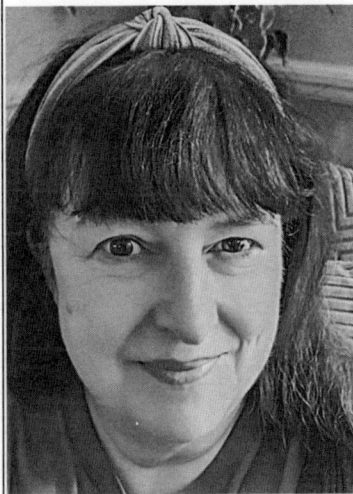

*Ellie Cadwallader White*

Four years ago, I was living in a body that felt more like a prison than a home. At size 32/34, I was unhealthy, unhappy and struggling to find any joy in life. I had completely given up on myself.

Food was my comfort and my punishment, and I had lost control over my eating, my body and my life. The scales ruled my days, dictating my mood and my self-worth, until, one day, I decided to pack them away for good.

Since then, I've dropped over 44kg (7st), but what's even more important is that I've regained control over my life. The scales no longer define me. My focus has shifted to feeling healthier and stronger, not chasing a number. I'm now wearing sizes 22, 20, and even 18, with a size 16 waiting in the wings, but these are just milestones on a much bigger journey. This journey is about reclaiming my life, my confidence and my happiness.

At 62, living with lipo-lymphoedema, traditional exercise like gym workouts or long walks isn't an option for me. But I still find ways to move more, in whatever way I can. Most of my progress has come from changing how I eat, making healthier choices that nourish my body rather than just filling it.

One of the most surprising victories for me has been the little things that most people take for granted. I can wear a belt now, paint my toenails without strain and get up from a chair without worrying if it'll stick to me. These small wins add up to a sense of control and freedom I hadn't felt in years.

To anyone starting their own journey or feeling a bit lost, my best advice is to relax and be patient. Quick fixes don't work. It's about playing the long game and understanding that setbacks are part of the process, not the end of the world.

The biggest change hasn't been in my dress size or even my weight. It's in how I see myself. I'm no longer the woman who had given up. I'm stronger, more confident and happier than I've been in years.

*Find out more about Ellie's story here:*

# CHAPTER 3

# Ending an Obsession
# With Food

Is food on your mind every waking hour? Do you find yourself obsessing over what you'll eat for your next meal while you're still at the table finishing your current one? Or perhaps you're branding foods relentlessly in your mind as 'good' and 'bad'?

If so, you're not alone. Food obsession is the third biggest psychological side effect of years of yo-yo dieting, according to 81 per cent of former dieters in my survey.

I've witnessed this happening to most people who have had a difficult relationship with food. In fact, the journey to sustainable weight loss is often marred by an overwhelming preoccupation with food – a phenomenon deeply rooted in our brain's mechanisms and psychological responses.

Why do our brains seem so fixated on food, especially when dieting? And what can be done about this obsession?

It's well documented that our brains are engineered for survival, compelling us to seek out and remember food sources, particularly those that provide quick energy such as fats and sugars.[1] This survival mechanism intensifies under food restriction, transforming mere food thoughts from necessity to an all-consuming fixation.[2]

For dieters, the journey often starts with self-imposed eating rules: what to eat, what not to eat and how much. Such restrictions can lead to feelings of deprivation, heightening the allure of 'forbidden' foods and often leading to the dreaded binge eating.[3] This forms a distressing cycle of restriction, obsession, overeating and guilt – starkly known as the 'rinse and repeat' cycle, impacting both mental and physical health.

This preoccupation isn't just a psychological phenomenon, but also has physiological roots, making food a central focus for those attempting to lose weight through strict dietary limitations.

When you embark on a calorie-restricted diet, the body perceives this as a signal of food scarcity, triggering a survival response designed to protect against starvation. The brain becomes hyper-alert to food-related cues, with thoughts of food becoming more persistent and intense. This response is not about willpower; it's a built-in biological mechanism geared towards survival.

From a psychological perspective, restrictive dieting can enhance the desirability of forbidden foods. The 'forbidden fruit' effect shows that when people are told to abstain from specific foods, their desire for these foods increases. A study in the journal *Appetite* demonstrated that people restricted from eating chocolate for a week had more intrusive thoughts about chocolate and a stronger urge to eat it compared to those not given the restriction.[4]

On the physiological side, dieting impacts levels of ghrelin and leptin, hormones that regulate hunger and satiety:

END AN OBSESSION WITH FOOD

- Ghrelin, known as the 'hunger hormone', increases with calorie restriction, signalling to the brain that it's time to eat.
- Leptin, which communicates satiety to the brain, drops when dieting, making you feel less full even after eating.

These two hormonal changes make dieters feel hungrier and, combined with the psychological impact of restriction, can lead to an obsession with food.[5]

Dieting primes your brain to focus on food. The constant thought of what you can and cannot eat keeps food at the forefront of your mind. This mental priming makes it difficult to escape food-related thoughts, resulting in an unhealthy preoccupation.

Embrace the strategies I've set out below with kindness and patience, and watch as you transform your approach to health and well-being into a more balanced, sustainable and fulfilling journey.

### How You Can Take Back Control

*Shift your mindset to nourishment*

Instead of focusing on what you can't eat, concentrate on what you can. Embrace a mindset of nourishment rather than deprivation. Choose foods that make you feel good and provide your body with the nutrients it needs. This positive focus can reduce the sense of restriction and help form a healthier relationship with food.

## Practise mindful eating

Mindful eating encourages paying attention to the experience of eating, savouring each bite and listening to your body's hunger and fullness cues. This practice can shift your focus from the quantity of food to the quality of the eating experience. A study showed that mindful eating can help reduce emotional eating and promote better self-regulation of food intake.[6]

## Aim for gradual change

Drastic weight loss is an unrealistic expectation. Celebrate small victories along the way to maintain motivation and avoid the all-or-nothing mindset that can lead to obsession.

## Limit exposure to food triggers

Reduce constant exposure to food-related stimuli that can prime the brain to focus on food. This might involve unfollowing social media accounts that emphasise dieting and food, or avoiding environments where you're likely to feel pressured to eat. Creating a supportive environment can help you stay focused on your overall health goals rather than being fixated on food.

Next, we're going to consider cravings, another psychological side effect of dieting, which you may be surprised to learn is very different from food obsession.

# Case Study: How I Took Back Control

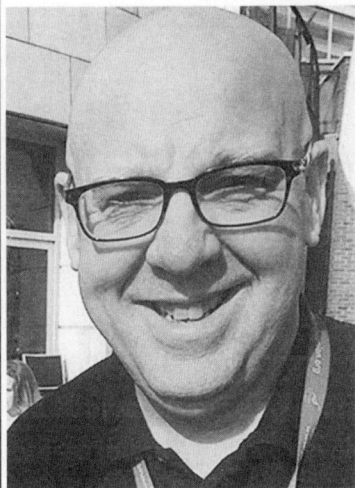

*Darin McCloud*

Probably the worst moment of my life was when I appeared in many of the national newspapers because I weighed over 125kg (20st) and had been told I'd have to put on more weight to qualify for a gastric band. I had a 122-cm (48-in) waist and type 2 diabetes – and I was desperate.

I used to eat non-stop. Food was the only thing on my mind. My main meals would consist of lots of takeaways and also cooked meals. While sometimes they were healthy, the portion sizes were large. I drank two litres of Coke a day (minimum) and crisps. I was always snacking on bread. At work, I'd go to the shops multiple times a day to buy pies, sandwiches, fish and chips, burgers and sweets. I was also depressed.

Luckily, Sandra saw my story and contacted me. She said she could help with her programme. That was 14 years ago. I couldn't believe how quickly things started changing. The biggest change was that I didn't miss Coke, sweets, chocolate bars and crisps. I then wanted to move more and my diabetes doctor suggested I start by running for a minute and walking for a minute.

Within six months, I ran the Great South Run, all

10k (6.2 miles) of it! I had lost 2.7kg (6lb) by then and had a 90-cm (36-in) waist! Afterwards I was walking on air.

I honestly can't believe the differences in my lifestyle in less than a year. Now I eat to fuel my body. I control food; food does not control me. I can eat what I choose, guilt-free, because my body tells me when I need to eat and, more importantly, when I've had enough. I exercise because it makes me feel good and I love it.

I've now run the London Marathon, cycled across Cuba and have won over 60 medals through running events. I also competed in a duathlon with double Olympic gold medallist Dame Kelly Holmes. And, to top it all off, I did an Ironman triathlon!

My blood sugar level went down so much my insulin dose was cut to zero, my body mass index (BMI) dropped a whole category and my depression lifted. At the Ironman weigh-in I was down to 92.5kg (14st 8lb) – meaning I'd lost over 36kg (80lb) since my unhappy days before Slimpod came into my life. I've kept all the weight off and life is fab.

If I can do it, anybody can!

*Find out more about Darin's story here:*

# CHAPTER 4

# Cravings: Dieting's Hidden Side Effect

Have you ever found yourself battling intense cravings while trying to stick to a diet?

Cravings are a common, and often frustrating, side effect of restrictive dieting, with 75 per cent surveyed in my Diet Dossier saying they experienced them.

Let's delve into the science behind cravings and explore practical ways to take back control. Understanding the underlying causes of cravings, including the brain's role and the psychological impact, can help you develop strategies to manage them effectively and maintain your weight-loss journey.

When you diet, your body and brain respond to perceived scarcity.[1] This response triggers powerful cravings for foods, particularly those high in sugar, fat and salt. These cravings are your body's age-old way of signalling a need for more energy and nutrients, designed to protect you from potential starvation.

Once again, the brain's reward system plays a crucial role in the formation and intensity of cravings. When you restrict your food intake, the brain becomes hypersensitive to food-related cues, making it harder to resist cravings.[2]

The anticipation and consumption of food, especially highly palatable foods, both release dopamine (see page 16). This process reinforces the desire to eat, making cravings more frequent and intense. Additionally, the prefrontal cortex – the part of the brain responsible for decision-making and impulse control – can become overworked and fatigued by constant dieting efforts, reducing its ability to regulate cravings effectively.

Research shows that we make around 200 food-related decisions every day.[3] Does it feel like that to you? Each decision requires willpower, and the more decisions you make, the more depleted your willpower becomes. As we'll see in Chapter 22, willpower operates on a limited reserve of mental energy, which depletes with use. This is known as decision fatigue.

Cravings can have a significant psychological impact, contributing to feelings of frustration, guilt and failure. When you give in to a craving, you might experience temporary relief followed by negative emotions, reinforcing a cycle of emotional eating. This cycle is often driven by cognitive biases, such as the 'all-or-nothing' mindset, where a single dietary slip is perceived as a complete failure. This mindset can lead to the 'what-the-hell' effect, where a minor lapse escalates into a full-blown binge (we'll explore this in more detail in Chapter 20). I bet sometimes you've said to yourself 'what the hell – I'll start again on Monday'! So many people have done this for so many years and it becomes a bad habit.

Research on self-regulation and eating behaviour explains how the 'what-the-hell' effect can exacerbate feelings of guilt and loss of control, further undermining dieting efforts.[4] Understanding these psychological dynamics is so important if you want to break the cycle and develop healthier eating habits. You *can* do it!

## How You Can Take Back Control

### Adopt a flexible eating approach

Instead of rigidly restricting certain foods, adopt a more flexible approach to eating. Allow yourself to enjoy a variety of foods in moderation, which can reduce the intensity of cravings. This approach, supported by research on intuitive eating, emphasises listening to your body's hunger and fullness cues, promoting a healthier relationship with food.[5]

### Be kind to yourself

When a craving arises, acknowledge it without judgement and remind yourself that it's okay to experience cravings. Research shows that self-compassion can reduce stress and promote healthier behaviours.[6] By being gentle with yourself, you can reduce the guilt and frustration that often accompany cravings and make more balanced choices.

### Question your hunger

Learn the difference between needing to eat to fuel your body and feeling you have to eat to satisfy an emotional need. Dampen down a craving by drinking a large glass of water. It really can work!

### Create a supportive environment

Modify your environment to support healthier eating habits and reduce exposure to food cues that trigger cravings.[7] This might involve keeping tempting foods out of sight, stocking your kitchen with healthy options and avoiding environments that promote unhealthy eating. Surround yourself with supportive people who encourage your health goals.

In the next chapter, we'll look at the way your mind lies to you about what you're capable of achieving and the negative effect these limiting self-beliefs can have on your attempts to lose weight.

# Case Study: How I Took Back Control

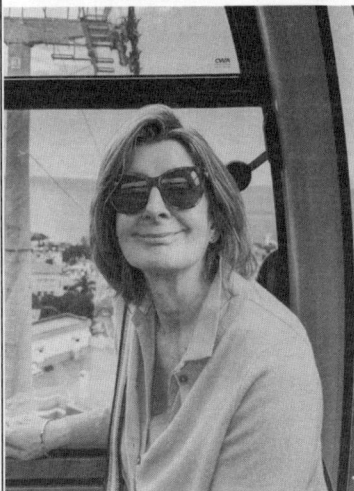

*Caroline R*

My problem was always consistency, balance and control. For years, I struggled with being overweight. I'd get motivated, work myself up and dive into a new diet. I'd lose some weight, but, as soon as I let my guard down, I'd revert to old habits and gain it all back. The mindset just wasn't right, and I could never maintain it. Life became a constant cycle of dieting, losing weight and then falling off the wagon.

My intentions were always good, but the balance was missing.

We've always eaten healthily; I've always cooked fresh meals. But my portions were too large. I'd heap my plate with pasta or other carbs until I felt uncomfortable. Late afternoons were especially tough. I'd hit a slump and crave sugar. If I came home from work as a nurse and found biscuits, I'd eat half the pack without a second thought. One or two would never be enough.

Everything changed after nine months on the Slimpod programme. Last Christmas, I still enjoyed all the festivities, but I didn't go overboard. I ate, drank and socialised without feeling restricted. The difference was I knew when I'd had enough. I could stop after one or two chocolates, knowing any more would make me feel terrible. It's completely transformed my approach to food.

By January, I was still the same weight I had been before Christmas. That was a first! We've had a few holidays since then and, again, it's all about balance. I enjoy the local food, but also make sure to stay active. A good walk every day is a must for me now. Otherwise, I just don't feel right.

My brain has finally balanced my whole food intake, and exercise has become crucial. My husband jokes that I'm a bit over the top about it, but I see it as essential. Just 30 minutes a day keeps me on track.

Now, if I come home hungry, I'll reach for something like wholemeal toast with peanut butter. I don't deprive myself, but I'm much more focused on nourishment.

Emotional eating used to be my downfall, especially when I was bored or upset. But I've gained confidence and control. Exercise boosts my mood, and I finally feel like I'm in charge of my life.

*Find out more about Caroline's story here:*

## CHAPTER 5

# Overcoming Self-Limiting Beliefs

Self-limiting beliefs are something we all accumulate during our lives and often they really hold us back from becoming the best version of ourselves. They're a huge factor in weight loss and at least one of these may seem familiar to you:

- 'I can't lose weight.'
- 'I can never keep the weight off.'
- 'I'm menopausal so can't lose weight.'
- 'I'm addicted to chocolate so will never lose weight.'
- 'I'm too old to shift the weight now.'

These statements are not true – they've all been made up by your mind, typically originating from a combination of personal experiences, deeply-ingrained thought patterns and societal influences.

Here's how they often develop:

### Past failures

Repeated attempts at losing weight that end in disappointment can lead to the formation of self-limiting beliefs. If you've tried various diets or exercise programmes without long-term success, it's easy to start believing that you're incapable of achieving your goals.[1] Each perceived failure chips away at your confidence, reinforcing the belief that you can't succeed.

## Negative feedback

Criticism from others, whether it's well-meaning or not, can significantly impact your self-perception.[2] Comments about your weight, appearance or eating habits can plant seeds of doubt and insecurity. Over time, these comments can grow into powerful self-limiting beliefs that undermine your efforts to change.

## Cultural and societal influences

Society often promotes unrealistic standards of beauty and fitness, especially on social media, which can create a sense of inadequacy. The pressure to conform to these standards can lead to the belief that you're not good enough or that you'll never achieve your ideal body. These societal messages can be pervasive and difficult to escape, reinforcing self-limiting beliefs.[3]

## Internal dialogue

The way you talk to yourself plays a crucial role in shaping your beliefs. Negative self-talk, such as calling yourself lazy or unworthy, can become a self-fulfilling prophecy. When you consistently tell yourself that you can't succeed, your actions and outcomes often align with that belief.[4]

Losing weight and improving your health is not just about changing your body; it's about changing your mind. Embrace the power you have within to redefine your beliefs and achieve your goals.

You deserve to feel confident, capable and empowered on your weight-loss journey. Let's make this transformation together, one positive thought at a time.

## How You Can Take Back Control

### Identify and challenge negative thoughts

The first step in reframing self-limiting beliefs is to identify them. Pay attention to the negative thoughts that pop into your mind, especially those related to your ability to lose weight. Once you've identified these thoughts, challenge them.

Ask yourself if they are based on facts or assumptions. For example, 'I'll never be able to lose 30 pounds' is an assumption, but 'I have been able to lose a few pounds in the past' is a fact. So lose a few pounds – which you know you can do – then concentrate on losing a few more, then a few more.

### Create positive affirmations

Affirmations are powerful statements that can help rewire your brain to think more positively. For example, instead of saying, 'I'll never lose weight,' try saying, 'I *am* capable of achieving my weight-loss goals.'

Repeat these affirmations daily, especially when you're feeling doubtful. Over time, these positive statements can help shift your mindset and build confidence.

## Focus on small wins

Celebrate small weight-loss victories. Did you choose a healthy meal over fast food? That's a win! Did you go for a walk instead of watching TV? Another win! Recognising and celebrating your progress, no matter how minor, can boost your confidence and reinforce positive beliefs about yourself.

These small successes add up and can help you see that you are capable of making positive changes.

## Mix with kind people

When you're surrounded by people who believe in you, it's easier to believe in yourself. Mix with those who uplift you and avoid those who bring you down.

# Case Study: How I Took Back Control

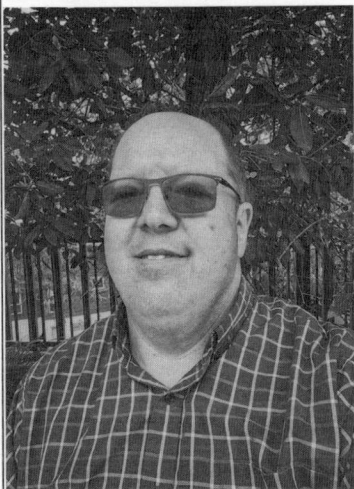

*John Burns*

My life had spiralled out of control, and I refused to recognise the person I'd become.

Some days after work, I'd reward myself for 'surviving' a nine-to-five day of home working with a large takeaway of Korean fried chicken. I'd conveniently ignore the fact that the restaurant had sent two sets of chopsticks because they assumed my order was for two people. On top of that, I'd order two cases of Pepsi Max with my weekly grocery delivery and often run out before the next delivery.

The wake-up call came last year during a business trip. I hadn't been on a plane for nearly a year and, when I tried to buckle my seatbelt, I realised I could barely get it done up. That was the moment I knew I needed to make a change, and fast.

I started looking online and stumbled across some ads on Facebook talking about mindset and healthy eating. The approach of the Slimpod programme intrigued me, so I decided to give it a shot.

The physical changes are great, of course. Trying on smaller clothes and finding they fit is a fantastic feeling. But, for me, this journey has been about trying

THE WEIGHT'S OVER

on new versions of myself. It's about realising that this isn't just a weight-loss programme – it's a self-development programme disguised as a weight-loss programme.

I've come to terms with the fact that I'd been holding on to limiting beliefs for a long time – beliefs that have held me back in ways I didn't even realise. I was used to wearing 2XL tops and size 40 trousers, and I was more than a little sceptical about whether anything could really help. But, within the first week, something incredible happened – my consumption of Pepsi Max dropped by 95 per cent. That was my first big win, and it felt amazing.

I've lost 15kg (2st 5lb) so far, and not only has my grocery shopping changed, but the frequency of my takeaway orders has decreased from twice a week to less than once a month. The journey isn't over, but, for the first time in my life, I feel like I'm truly in control.

*Find out more about John's story here:*

• 38 •

## CHAPTER 6

# The Hidden Impact of Dieting on Self-Esteem

When you start out on a restrictive diet, you might think you're taking control of your health and your body. But what often gets overlooked is how diets can damage your self-esteem. The constant battle to control your calorie intake can lead to feelings of failure and inadequacy.

You've probably done umpteen diets – my Diet Dossier survey showed that 39 per cent of people had been on 15 or more diets – so I'm sure you recognise this feeling: on day one of a new diet there's a sense of relief that finally you're taking charge of your life. The tiny bit of scepticism at the back of your mind – 'Nothing's ever worked before so why is this going to be different?' – is swept aside the moment you drop the first pound or two. Suddenly, your confidence and self-esteem get a much-needed boost.

Here's the downside: research shows that restrictive diets often lead to overeating and binge-eating episodes.[1] When the diet inevitably fails and the weight comes back, it's easy to feel like you've failed.

This cycle of weight loss and gain (what a lot of people know as yo-yo dieting) can erode your self-esteem, making you feel inadequate and convincing you you're incapable of achieving your goals. Studies have found that chronic dieters often experience lower self-esteem than non-dieters.[2] The constant cycle of diet-fail-diet-fail reinforces negative self-talk and the self-limiting beliefs we explored in the previous chapter, leading to a diminished self-image.

When you regain the weight you worked so hard to lose, it's common to blame yourself. This self-blame can spiral into a negative mindset, further damaging your self-esteem.

One problem we all face is that, in our Western society, thinness is often idolised and dieting is seen as the path to achieving this ideal. Social media and advertising bombard us with images of 'perfect' bodies, setting unrealistic standards. A thought-provoking piece of research done back in the 1950s explains how we determine our worth in all aspects of life by comparing ourselves to others.[3] This constant comparison can lead to feelings of inadequacy and lower self-esteem when you feel you don't measure up.

It has been shown that exposure to media images of thin people significantly increases body dissatisfaction among women.[4] This grows the more you constantly strive for an often unattainable ideal. And there's a harmful knock-on effect: the pressure to conform to these beauty standards can lead to you equating your worth as a parent, partner or person with your ability to achieve a certain body type. I know from my own teenage years how painful and damaging that can be.

Dieting can also lead to something called cognitive dissonance, a psychological phenomenon where you experience mental discomfort because how you want to behave conflicts with your deep-rooted beliefs (we'll explore cognitive dissonance in more detail in Chapter 21).

You have two choices to reduce the discomfort: change how you behave or change what you believe.[5] If you're trying to lose weight, then you change the behaviour by eating high-calorie food; or you change your beliefs by being negative and telling yourself, 'Oh well, it was never going to work' or, worse, 'I'm just a hopeless case and I always fail.' Bang goes your self-esteem.

By being aware of the impact of dieting on your self-esteem, you can take steps to protect and improve your self-worth because, in my experience, this is at the root of so much comfort eating. I absolutely love it when I see people start to break free from their limitations and begin to become the best version of themselves. They then naturally take back control of food in the process – wonderful!

Remember – you absolutely can feel confident, capable and empowered on your weight-loss journey; it's totally possible and you deserve it!

## How You Can Take Back Control

*Blame dieting, not yourself*

Now you know how much the brain's reaction to dieting can hammer your self-esteem, stop doing yourself down all the time. Forget about your weight and concentrate on things that really make you feel good, like long walks and relaxing hot baths.

*Being kind really works*

Your weight-loss journey will always hit a few bumps in the road. Small setbacks aren't disasters, so give yourself a break. Research shows that self-compassion is linked to higher self-esteem and emotional resilience.[6]

*Challenge negative thoughts*

Take a deep breath and count to five. Taking a pause can stop the thought from spiralling. Challenge it by asking, 'Is this thought really true?' You'll often find your negative thought is based more on feelings than facts. Replace it with a positive affirmation.

*Limit social media*

Cut down your exposure to social media and advertising that promotes unrealistic body standards. Follow people and products that are body positive and recognise that true beauty is on the inside. Focus on your unique strengths and accomplishments rather than comparing yourself to others.

## Case Study: How I Took Back Control

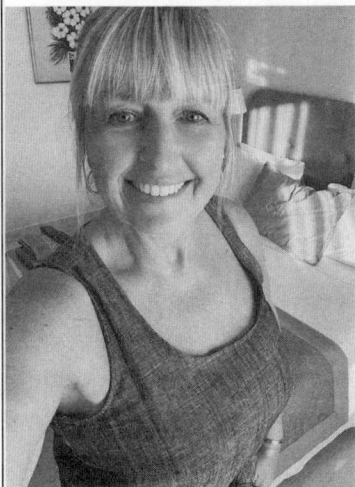

*Lynn Haddrell*

For over 40 years, I lived with guilt and shame around food. I can still vividly remember being a young child and asking for a biscuit. My mum got cross and said no because I couldn't possibly be hungry, even though I was. She constantly made comments that I was a 'big girl' for my age or that I was getting fat.

From that moment, food became a source of guilt for me. I started avoiding second helpings or so-called 'bad foods', even when I was still hungry, because I was afraid of being judged. But that didn't stop the feelings of hunger and desire for comfort. That's when the secret eating began.

I would spend all my pocket money on sweets and chocolate and gobble them up in secret. They comforted me, and no one could judge me if they didn't know. But, of course, the guilty feelings just got worse.

As I grew up, the toxic relationship I had with food continued. I lost count of how many diets I tried and failed. Some worked temporarily – I'd reach my goal weight through sheer deprivation – but then I'd revert to secret eating and bingeing. The weight would pile back on, and the cycle of shame would begin again.

All of that ended for me when I discovered how

Slimpod could help me transform my mindset. Today, after decades of dieting, I'm finally free and haven't dieted for four years. My brain has stopped labelling food as good or bad, which wasn't helpful. Food is just food, and I now get to choose what to eat and when.

I no longer eat in secret, and I've detached all those feelings of guilt and shame from food. Now, I mostly choose to eat healthily, but it's because I want to, not because I feel like I have to.

I've been able to unpick all the difficult and painful beliefs I had held on to for years. I've learned to work through my emotions instead of suppressing them with comfort food. I'm now a normal eater with a healthy relationship with food and with myself. I'm free from the mental prison I'd built for myself.

This journey is about so much more than becoming physically smaller. It's about growing in ways I never dreamed possible. Four years ago, I was embarrassed by my size and how unfit I was. I was clinically depressed and terrified of getting old. Today, I've walked on fire, taken up tennis and yoga, completed a 5-k (3.1-mile) obstacle course and climbed Glastonbury Tor without needing an ambulance.

I've learned to be my own cheerleader and, finally, I make no apologies for being me.

*Find out more about Lynn's story here:*

# CHAPTER 7

# Breaking Through Fear: Your Path to Success

Does this sound familiar? You've been making great progress on your weight-loss journey. You've developed healthy eating habits, committed to regular exercise and are feeling fantastic. Then suddenly, out of nowhere, you hit a wall. It's as if a light in your brain has been switched off. The motivation that once fuelled your every step vanishes, replaced by a creeping sense of dread. Fear of failure rears its ugly head, and you find yourself paralysed, worrying that all your hard-earned progress is slipping away.

If this sounds familiar, rest assured you're not alone. In my Diet Dossier survey, more than half the people said they had suffered from it. It's not just fear of failure that can act as a significant barrier on your path to a healthier lifestyle but also, strangely, the fear of success. Both fears are deeply rooted in your past experiences with dieting and food, often leading to the self-limiting beliefs we explored in Chapter 5 that hold you back from achieving your goals.

Studies have shown that the fear of regaining weight can be even more stressful than the initial weight-loss journey itself, leading to a cycle of fear that hampers further progress.[1]

These fears are exacerbated by settings such as slimming clubs where public weigh-ins can evoke feelings of humiliation or judgement if progress doesn't meet expectations. The constant worry about not only losing weight but also maintaining the loss can lead to what psychologists call 'anticipatory anxiety', where the fear of a potential outcome becomes a self-fulfilling prophecy.[2]

The psychological impact of this fear is profound. It often leads to avoidance behaviours; instead of pushing through the fear, you might avoid situations where failure could occur, like skipping weigh-ins or abandoning healthy eating and exercise routines altogether.[3]

It's important to recognise that fear is a normal emotional response, not a sign of weakness. Fear uses our past to shape our expectations of the future, often inaccurately. By understanding its roots and mechanisms, and by actively employing strategies to combat it, you can continue your journey towards a healthier future without being held back by the past. It involves a conscious effort to confront and reframe our fears.

Encouragingly, research suggests that behavioural strategies which help individuals challenge and change their thought patterns can be particularly effective in addressing the fear of failure.[4]

Remember, every step forward, no matter how small, is a victory over fear.

## How You Can Take Back Control

*Challenge your fears*

Recognise that deep-rooted fear of failure in weight loss is a powerful but surmountable barrier. Challenge catastrophic thoughts about failure by questioning their validity. Replace 'My partner will leave me if I don't lose 15kg' with 'My partner loves me because of the person I am.' Fears are not facts. They're a fiction about the future.

*Set achievable goals*

Chunk down your weight-loss journey into small, manageable goals. Aiming to lose 0.5kg (1lb) a week seems a breeze compared to losing 23kg (50lb) in a year, so boost your confidence and reduce the pressure on yourself by setting tinier targets.

*Cultivate resilience*

Make every day have meaning. Do something that gives you a sense of success and purpose so you don't dwell on your fears. Learn from the past and how you coped with tough times then. Always say 'I can' not 'I can't.'

# Case Study: How I Took Back Control

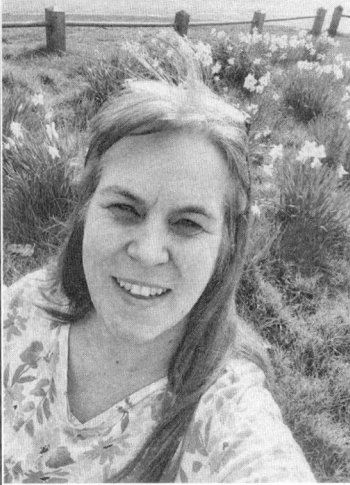

*Colette Molloy*

As a biologist, I knew the theory behind healthy living, yet I couldn't recognise the damage I was doing to my own body. I was caught in a toxic cycle – starving myself with restrictive diets only to give in to cravings and binge on high-fat, sugar-laden foods. In hindsight, the most ridiculous part was that my fear of damaging my body led to me scrimping on nutritious meals to save 'points' for unhealthy snacks like crisps and sweets. I was starving my body of the nutrients it needed, poisoning it with sugar and chemicals. My eating habits became increasingly emotional, and I turned to convenience foods for comfort. Looking back, I realise I was self-harming with food.

In the summer of 2021, I was diagnosed with hypothyroidism and fatty liver infiltration. The liver issue, I knew, was due to my carb-heavy diet. My GP's advice was the same as always: lose weight and avoid alcohol, despite the fact I rarely drank. I felt frustrated and lost.

A friend introduced me to Slimpod and, after my first listen, I was suddenly conscious of my food choices. Almost overnight, my emotional bingeing stopped. Something changed mentally – I was filled with hope and belief, not fear.

I started cooking meals from scratch, using real ingredients. Batch-cooking became my norm, and I organised my vegetables for quick meals after work instead of reaching for ready meals. The weight started to drop, but this time it felt different. I didn't feel like I was on a wagon that I could fall off; everything felt natural and sustainable.

Then, I went through a break-up. In the past, that would have derailed me completely, but I didn't lose focus. A month later, I was diagnosed with breast cancer. I was devastated. After making all these healthy changes, it felt so unfair. Now I had a new fear to deal with. My consultants warned me about potential weight gain from the treatments, but I was determined not to let that happen. Even through the hardest parts of my treatment, I stuck to my healthy habits and continued to lose weight.

By the following July, I achieved my goal of fitting into a size 12 dress, down from a size 20 in January. After a year of treatment, I was stunned to find I'd lost 25kg (4st). A fellow Slimpodder encouraged me to enter the London Moonwalk for breast cancer. I completed the 26.2-mile walk and even did it again this year, despite limited training.

Now, I feel empowered. My GP recently confirmed that both my fatty liver and hypothyroidism have reversed – an incredible win. My life has transformed, and I'm finally living it to the fullest.

*Find out more about Colette's story here:*

# PART TWO

# Everything's Been Stacked Against You

It's vital to understand that if you've tried to lose weight but have never succeeded, it's not your fault. Your brain, the food you eat and the kind of world you live in have all been conspiring to make you fail. Here's what you need to know to take back control.

# CHAPTER 8

# Factory Food Is Making the World Fatter

If you've got an old family photo album, look at the pictures of your grandparents and your parents when they were young. Chances are you'll be surprised to see that they all look slim and healthy. Being overweight is a fairly recent phenomenon and research puts the blame on the ultra-processed food we eat, produced in factories not fields.[1]

The statistics show that, in the UK, men put on only about 7kg (15lb) between 1938 and 1968. By 1968, Mr Average weighed 72kg (159lb). By 1993 he had grown to 79kg (174lb). Head forward 30 years to the present and he weighs 85.4kg (188lb).[2] **Ask yourself why.**

In 1968, the average British woman was 157.50cm (5ft 2in) tall, weighed 61.6kg (136lb), had size three feet and was a dress size 12. Today she weighs 70kg (155lb). So the average woman in 2025 weighs only a few pounds less than the average man did in 1968! What's really noticeable is just how much bra sizes have increased: 60 years ago, women were 34B on average but today they're 36DD. **Again, ask yourself why.**

In the United States, the average man weighed 77kg (170lb) in 1962 and the average woman weighed 67kg (148lb). Today, the average American man weighs 90kg (199lb) and the average woman weighs 77kg (171lb).[3] **Once more, ask yourself why.**

Clearly something has slowly been making us all put on weight. And like so many things that changed our lives in Britain, it all began in America.

In the late 1940s, various studies showed a link between high-fat diets and high cholesterol levels, and suggested that a low-fat diet might be healthier. The trouble was, there was no clear evidence that a low-fat diet prevented heart disease or promoted weight loss.[4]

In the 1960s, the notion of dieting – using willpower to starve yourself of calories, especially carbohydrates and fat – took hold. Then in the 1970s and into the 80s, low-fat became an all-powerful ideology wholeheartedly backed by governments, doctors, food makers and the media. Millions bought anything labelled 'low fat' without a second thought about what other ingredients it might contain, such as sugar, which is four times as addictive as cocaine.[5]

Let me repeat that in case you thought your eyes were deceiving you: research shows that sugar is four times as addictive as cocaine. And yet the food industry has been packing us with sugar for more than half a century.

Here's the great irony of the low-fat obsession: while many people were drastically reducing their fat intake and starving themselves on diets, they just kept getting fatter and fatter. They were brainwashed to ignore the evidence in front of their eyes. They were led to believe that fat was the major cause of them gaining weight and 'low fat' helped them lose it. But it was a myth; actually, a downright lie.

Because low-fat products nearly always have a higher sugar content.[6]

Today, we face an even bigger menace. Once our food came fresh, straight from the farm; now it comes ultra-processed, straight from the factory. The makers call it convenience food; I call it fake food.

It seems that few people make the connection between obesity and the hidden sugar in ultra-processed food such as ready meals, takeaways, pizzas, pies and fizzy drinks. Yet, all the time, the culprit is there to be seen in the list of ingredients on every packet, jar, can and bottle: high fructose corn syrup (HFCS for short).

It never occurred to anyone that all those giant helpings of fizzy colas, massively laced with HFCS, might be the catalyst for harmful bodily change. Why would they? Their thinking was that there was no fat in fizzy drinks, so how could it be bad for them?

Here's the science: fructose does not stimulate insulin secretion or enhance leptin production – hormones which are vital to balancing your body weight. Because insulin and leptin act as key signals in the regulation of food intake and body weight, this suggests that dietary fructose may contribute to increased calorie intake and weight gain.[7]

In plain English, they make you want to eat more and more, leading to overconsumption. Your full signal is overridden and it becomes impossible to resist the sweet stuff in ever-increasing quantities. The more you eat and drink, the more you want. Scientists know that fructose triggers cravings for fatty foods and carbohydrates, while blocking the body's ability to use stored energy in fat.[8] That's a scary light-bulb moment.

In America, the consumption of HFCS increased more than 1,000 per cent between 1970 and 1990, far exceeding the changes in intake of any other food or food group. HFCS now represents more than 40 per cent of sweeteners added to food and beverages and is the sole sweetener in soft drinks in the United States.[9]

Why is what happens in America so important for the rest of the Western world? Because many of us are subconsciously driven to copy what goes on across the Atlantic. The subliminal brainwashing happens mainly through TV and films; we see apparently affluent Americans enjoying fast food, takeaways and gigantic colas and we want to be like them. And as we get bigger, we even start to dress like them in baggy T-shirts and shorts.

Look at any high street in Britain today and you'll see an abundance of American food outlets: McDonald's, Burger King, KFC, Subway . . . the list is endless. Visit a shopping centre and the chances are you'll eat in that other American invention, the food court. We're becoming more Americanised every day.

Everywhere you look, food is being pushed at you in irresistible and glamorised ways. On supermarket shelves, glossy packaging lures you to take home ready meals and treats for the kids. Every ad break on TV seems to be all about food, much of it delivered direct to your door. Fortunes are spent producing slick TV ads which promote the feeling that food makes families happy. Is it any wonder we're all eating more and more? Who wouldn't want to be happy?

Wrong question. What we should be asking is: Who wants to be healthy? Because living on a constant diet of sugar-packed, processed food is a recipe for disaster. Umpteen research studies suggest a strong link between excess sugar intake and diabetes, heart disease and certain cancers.[10] One leading food expert, Dr Chris van Tulleken, associate professor at University College London, has gone so far as to claim that processed food manufacturers pose as big a risk to public health as tobacco companies by selling addictive products that could be harmful.[11]

When you add it all up – the fake news about low fat, the food manufacturers turning you into sugar addicts, the pressure of TV advertising, the inexorable rise of fattening junk food – one thing shouts out loud and clear: IT'S NOT YOUR FAULT!

I can't repeat this often enough. For all your life, everything has been stacked against you and it's gradually getting worse. If you're determined to lose weight but can't, I make no apology for yelling this important fact once again: IT'S NOT YOUR FAULT!

So be kind to yourself. Give yourself a break. Positivity is a vital building block in retraining your brain to be on your side, not working against you.

## How You Can Take Back Control

I asked bestselling author and nutritionist Rob Hobson to tell us a bit more about UPFs and his top tips to reduce their impact. This is what he said:

*Why do UPFs contribute to weight gain and how can you cut them down in your diet?*
I think it's safe to assume we have all heard about UPFs and how they are affecting our health. These foods are a key focus of conversation around body weight and the rising global rates of obesity as UPFs now dominate modern diets. There has been a lot of focus on specific ingredients like additives, but these are still under scrutiny and the real concern lies in the overall structure of UPFs and their inescapable availability in the modern food environment. The issue is not just in the ingredients themselves, but the way UPFs are engineered to promote overconsumption while lacking essential nutrients.

*What does the research say about UPFs and body weight?*
There is now a large body of research showing a direct association between high intake of UPFs and increased BMI. The ease of access, affordability and ubiquity of UPFs make them a staple in many diets, particularly among people with limited food budgets. While socio-economic status and physical activity levels contribute to obesity, UPFs significantly influence how much food we eat, the nutrients we get from food and weight gain.

## Why are UPFs associated with overweight and obesity?

UPFs are often consumed more quickly due to their soft textures and lack of fibre, which contributes to a higher intake of calories, and their addictive nature and convenience make it easier for individuals to consume more than they need. However, while some evidence suggests that faster eating rates are linked to overeating, not all UPFs contribute to this pattern, such as 'healthier' UPFs including high-fibre bread products and plant-based ready-prepared foods made with legumes.

## What other factors are involved?

- **Hyper-palatability:** UPFs are engineered to appeal to our taste buds by combining added sugars, fats and salt in a way that stimulates the brain's reward system, leading to overeating even when you're not hungry.
- **Food access and cost:** UPFs are often more accessible and affordable than whole foods, especially in low-income areas, and their convenience and long shelf life make them easy choices for many people.
- **Blood sugar:** The refined carbohydrates and added sugars in UPFs can cause rapid spikes and dips in blood sugar, leading to cycles of hunger and overeating.
- **Gut health and microbiome:** Some research suggests that UPFs may impact on the gut microbiome, which in turn could be linked to obesity via the regulation of hunger, increased energy harvested from food by certain bacteria and chronic inflammation. While the relationship

between UPFs and gut health is not fully understood, altered gut microbiota is increasingly being linked to obesity and metabolic disorders.

## Why are UPFs addictive?

The combination of sugar, fat and salt in UPFs activates the brain's reward centres, similar to addictive substances, triggering the release of dopamine. This can lead to a cycle of craving and reward, where people seek out UPFs for comfort or as a coping mechanism, which can result in eating too much and putting on weight.

UPFs are associated with increased calorie intake and obesity, but the underlying mechanisms are complex. More research is needed to fully understand how UPFs impact appetite, digestion and metabolism, but the growing body of evidence suggests that reducing UPF consumption is a key step in maintaining a healthy body weight. Eliminating UPFs completely from the diet is not as simple as it sounds and unachievable for many people. A better approach is to shift the focus towards including more unprocessed foods in your diet rather than fixating on what you should be excluding from your diet.

## Eight simple tips to reduce your intake of UPFs

1. **Assess your current diet:** Review what you're eating and what's in your kitchen to gauge your UPF intake. This will help you plan your approach.
2. **Identify your weakest point:** Pinpoint when you're most likely to reach for UPFs (for example, at work lunches, post-work meals) and tackle this first. Prepare simple

alternatives like cooked chicken with salad or batch-cook easy dinners like chilli or Bolognese.

3. **Keep it simple:** Mealtimes don't need to be complicated, so keep a repertoire of quick-fix recipes like scrambled egg or omelette, tinned tuna salad, roast salmon and vegetables or tofu stir-fry.

4. **Get organised:** Organisation is key so plan and get everything in stock to create easy meals throughout the week. Batch-cook and freeze a few dishes so there is always something to hand when you really don't feel like cooking.

5. **Create a healthy food environment:** The UPF food environment can be really challenging when you are trying to lose weight, so don't recreate it at home. Try to keep UPF snacks out of the kitchen, so they are viewed more as an occasional food rather than an everyday staple.

6. **Shop wisely:** Some store-bought products are better than others. Learn to read labels to choose options with fewer additives, but don't forget to also keep looking at the traffic light labels on the front of pack to help guide your food choices – it's not all the about additives.

7. **Choose the lesser of two UPFs:** If you can't avoid UPFs entirely, choose the product with the simplest ingredient list.

8. **Start simple and get the family involved:** Involve your family in cooking and start with easy recipes. Shop locally for cost-effective ingredients to make cooking from scratch budget-friendly.

Let's now look at some more weight issues that also aren't your fault. Then we'll work out what you can do about them.

## CHAPTER 9

# The Hidden Hurdle of Addictions

Is this you? You're totally committed to your goal of lasting weight loss, but you find yourself constantly battling intense cravings for sugary snacks, comfort foods or that nightly glass of wine. These cravings feel overpowering, almost as if they have a mind of their own. This isn't a sign of weak willpower or lack of discipline; it's the hallmark of addiction, and it can make weight loss feel like an insurmountable challenge.

Addictions to food, sugar and alcohol are more common than you might think, and they play a significant role in why many people struggle to lose weight and keep it off. To understand how to overcome these addictions, it's crucial to look at the science behind them and how our brains are intricately involved in the process.

Addiction is a complex condition that affects the brain's reward system, which we met on page 15. It begins with a behaviour that provides a rewarding or pleasurable experience. This can be anything from eating a sugary treat to drinking alcohol. The brain responds to these pleasurable experiences by releasing dopamine. Over time, the brain starts to crave these experiences, and the behaviours become habitual.

Scientific research has shown that food addiction, particularly to sugar, triggers the same brain pathways as addictive drugs like cocaine and heroin. One study demonstrated that sugar bingeing releases dopamine in the brain's reward centres, similar to drug addiction.[1] This dopamine release reinforces the behaviour, making it more likely that you'll seek out sugary foods again to replicate the pleasurable feeling. But the effect soon wears off. Each time, the dopamine hit becomes less potent, leading you to seek more of what gave you the buzz in the first place.[2]

Alcohol addiction follows a similar pathway. When you drink alcohol, it increases the release of dopamine, giving you a feeling of euphoria. However, over time, the brain becomes less sensitive to dopamine, requiring more alcohol to achieve the same pleasurable effect.[3]

One of the most challenging aspects of addiction is that it alters the brain's structure and function. Prolonged exposure to addictive substances, whether they are food, sugar, drugs or alcohol, changes the way the brain processes rewards and self-control. This is why breaking free from any addiction is not just a matter of willpower; it's about rewiring the brain. It gives me the biggest thrill every day when I see people take back control!

The prefrontal cortex (see page 28) is particularly affected by addiction. Studies have shown that individuals with addictions have reduced activity in the prefrontal cortex, making it harder for them to resist cravings and make healthy choices.[4]

Understanding the role of the brain in addiction helps explain why it's so difficult to overcome these cravings. It's not just about resisting the compulsive urge to eat a doughnut or have a glass of wine; it's about changing the way your brain responds to these triggers.

By incorporating the strategies that follow into your daily routine, you can start to break free from the grip of addiction and support your weight-loss journey. It's important to remember that overcoming addiction is a process, and it's okay to seek help and support along the way. Talk to your health professional about what's available.

## How You Can Take Back Control

*Think before you eat*

Become more aware of your cravings and think about what triggers them. Gradually learn to observe your cravings without acting on them. Use all your senses to savour smaller portions, eating slowly and chewing every morsel.

*Healthy substitutes*

If you crave sugary snacks, try eating fruit or nuts instead. If you usually have a glass of wine in the evening, try drinking a herbal tea or sparkling water with a splash of fruit juice. By replacing unhealthy habits with healthier ones, you can start to rewire your brain's reward system.

*Support and counselling*

Talking to others who are going through similar struggles can help you feel less alone and more motivated to stay on track. CBT is particularly effective for treating addiction, as it helps you identify and change negative thought patterns and behaviours.[5]

*Physical activity*

Regular exercise increases the release of endorphins, which are natural mood boosters. Exercise also helps regulate dopamine levels in the brain, reducing the need for addictive substances.[6]

In the next chapter, I'm going to reveal something you'll wish you'd known for years: the science that shows how dieting makes weight loss harder.

## Case Study: How I Took Back Control

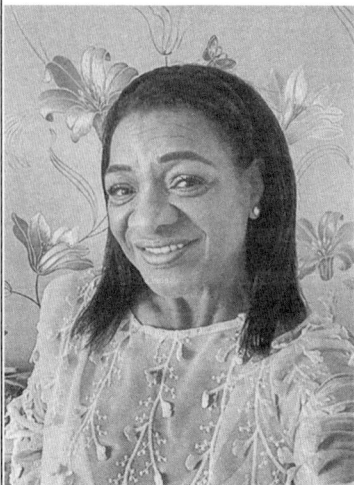

*Ava Brodie*

Ever since I was a girl, I'd had a sweet tooth. I can't remember a day going by without eating sweet stuff – I was a sugarholic. But it's important to realise it's never too late to take your health back and, when I finally understood the harm sugar was doing to my body, I decided it was time to change.

Slimpod gave me the power to be able to do that. So I went cold turkey and stopped having sugar overnight. For the first ten days I had side effects: headaches, spots and rashes on my face, sleep disruptions, fatigue, irritability and cravings for carbohydrates!

Then, after that, I started to feel so much better. I had more energy, better quality of sleep, a clearer complexion, a feeling of contentment – and no more sweet cravings! What helped me was drinking two litres of water a day, eating protein with each meal, eating more berries and citrus fruit, and replacing coffee with hot water and a slice of lemon, or green tea.

After one week of going sugar-free my weight started to come off and I lost 16kg (36lb) in the first six months. I feel more energised and happier than I have in a long time. To be finally free from sugar is such a relief.

Apart from being healthier, the other bonus is that I've dropped from a size 16 to a size 8 and I've lost 10cm (4in) from my waistline. My BMI has dropped from 29.5 to 23.5 – which means that I'm no longer overweight, let alone being on the verge of obesity.

Slimpod made me realise I *can* stop eating sugar. My mindset is stronger than ever, no more diet mentality, and I no longer have any issue with sugar.

I now believe in myself and know that these healthy new habits are so ingrained that I will have them for life.

*Find out more about Ava's story here:*

## CHAPTER 10

# Why Dieting Makes Weight Loss Harder

Losing weight and keeping it off can feel like an uphill battle. You might wonder why it's so tough, especially if you've spent so many years on yo-yo diets. The truth is, there's a lot going on in your mind and body that makes maintaining weight loss challenging.

Researchers have found that most people who lose weight by dieting regain about 30–35 per cent of it within the first year, and up to 50 per cent within 5 years.[1] This can happen even for people who've had weight-loss surgery.

It's not about failing or giving up; it's about how your body responds to weight loss. Only by retraining your brain so your mind and body work hand in hand can you hope to lose weight in a sustainable way.

When weight isn't an issue, hormones from your gut, pancreas and fat tissues are constantly signalling your brain to regulate how much you eat and how much energy you burn. However, when you lose weight by dieting, your body kicks in several mechanisms to bring the weight back. Crucial hormones change in ways that make you hungrier and slow down your metabolism, making it easier to regain weight.

A landmark study showed what happens to your hormones when you lose weight and try to keep it off.[2] Participants followed a low-calorie diet for 10 weeks and lost about 13.5kg (30lb). Researchers measured their levels of various hormones before, during and after the diet and found that the levels of hormones that make you feel full, like leptin, peptide YY, cholecystokinin, insulin and amylin, decreased. At the same time, levels of the hunger hormone ghrelin increased, and participants felt hungrier. A year later, these hormonal changes and increased hunger persisted.

Your genes play a significant part in your weight, too. Large-scale studies have shown that there are almost 150 genetic variants linked to obesity.[3] Even after you lose weight, your genes might be pushing you back towards your higher weight. The fact is your body has a set point it wants to return to, and half of it is genetics and half environment.

We all have a biological survival mechanism that conserves energy in the face of starvation and dangerously low energy supplies. It's called adaptive thermogenesis, which is a fancy way of describing the slowing of your metabolic rate as a response to weight loss. In America, 16 contestants on the TV show *The Biggest Loser* took part in a scientific study.[4] Their weight, body composition and metabolic rate were measured at the end of the competition and again six years later. The participants had all rapidly lost massive amounts of weight on the show, but were found to have regained most with time. The winner of the competition lost 108kg (239lb) but six years later had put 45kg (100lb) back on. Thirteen of the contestants regained all or most of their weight in six years. Four were heavier than before the competition. There was only one contestant who weighed less than she did at the end of the competition.

Human biology is a powerful driver of weight regain, so maintaining weight lost by dieting, without retraining the brain to have a different relationship with food, will always be a challenge.

There are many other reasons why people regain weight after losing it. Obesity often comes with a strong preference for tasty, high-fat and high-sugar foods. When you cut these out, you can experience cravings, fatigue and a bad mood. Losing weight also affects the brain's pleasure centres. You get less reward from eating driven by dopamine. This lack of pleasure can make you eat more to try to feel good again (see Chapter 9).

By understanding these biological changes, you can better tackle the challenges of maintaining weight loss and work towards a more sustainable, healthier lifestyle.

## How You Can Take Back Control

I asked Dale Pinnock, TV's Medicinal Chef, to tell us a bit more about what different food types do to our bodies and to give us his top tips on eating a balanced diet:

It is fair to say that, when it comes to long-term diets and healthy eating patterns, so many of us are completely and utterly confused, and when we look at the vast amount of chatter about diet in the media, is it any wonder? There are so many different diets and approaches to eating out there. Which is right? Which should we follow?

Well, ultimately, there are grains of truth in almost all of these different dietary patterns, but are these approaches sustainable in the long term? No! There always seems to be some kind of restriction or removal of a food group, or strange habit that we need to adopt. Sure, it may give you some short-term results, but what about the long game? What can you do for a lifetime that is actually easy, sustainable and enjoyable, and will deliver long-term health benefits and help to protect you from the many diet and lifestyle diseases that plague us in this part of the world? Well, thankfully, it is actually very simple.

There are a few key guidelines you can follow to build a healthful way of eating for a lifetime – all based on the totality of the science, and all really simple. Have these few guidelines in mind and you will never go far wrong:

### Swap the white for the brown

One of the big keys for a long-term healthy diet is the type of carbohydrates we are consuming. This simple tip – swap your white for brown – will seriously move the health needle in the right direction. In the modern world we are eating far too many processed carbohydrates such as white bread, white rice, white pasta and, of course, the obvious sweets and sugary foods. The issue with these foods is that they release their glucose content rapidly. This in turn sends blood sugar up very high very quickly. Now, of course, blood sugar rises after eating. It is supposed to. The issue is how far it rises and how rapidly, and the metabolic knock-on effects that follow such an aggressive rise. If we eat some of these foods now and again and get such a response, then it is of absolutely no consequence to the body whatsoever. But, if we eat these things three times a day every day (think toast at breakfast, a sandwich at lunch, and so on . . . it soon adds up), then the constant aggressive sugar increases start to cause problems. It can raise our cholesterol (yep, as much as the wrong fats can), it can increase abdominal weight gain that is hard to shift and it can increase risk of type 2 diabetes. Not to mention age our skin faster and increase inflammation in the body. Now, it is *not* carbohydrates doing this. It is the rate and the extent to which blood sugar rises in a short space of time, and the biochemical chaos this causes that is driving these issues. If we change our carb choices, we take away the issue. How do we do that? We swap the white for the brown. If you swap white rice for brown rice, white bread for brown bread, and so on, then you have staple carbs that have just as much glucose in them as the white variety, but they have something the white ones don't – they have fibre! Fibre makes these carb sources far harder to digest, which in turn means their glucose content is liberated far more slowly. This leads to blood sugar that rises gently and slowly, which does not give us any of the metabolic and hormonal disaster that follows aggressive spikes. Plus you get sustained energy levels, and these higher fibre varieties contain far more micronutrients such as B vitamins, zinc and selenium to boot, too!

## Always think: 'Where is the protein?'

Now, this doesn't mean I am going to tell you to go all cave dweller. But, whenever you look at your plate, once you have the high-fibre, slow-burning carbs ticked off, the next inclusion needs to be a protein source. Absolutely, this could be meat or fish, but it could also be eggs, beans and pulses, tofu, tempeh . . . whatever your preferences are. The reason this is important is that this will further add to the blood sugar stabilisation effect. When you add protein to a high-fibre carb source, you create a meal that takes far more digestive effort to break down, which leads to further slowing of blood sugar rises, meaning more stable energy levels, less brain fog and, of course, less risk of those issues that I described above. Plus, of course, the more diversity on your plate, the more diversity of nutrients. This leads me nicely on to the next fundamental . . .

## Always ensure a diversity of plant foods

Plants rule the roost when it comes to a healthy dietary pattern for the long term. I am not saying go vegan, but I am saying that plants need to dominate your plate – at every meal. Whether that is berries with your porridge or indeed fresh fruit throughout the morning; a good varied side salad with your lunch – think baby spinach, red peppers, beetroot, red onions, not just some limp iceberg lettuce; or a variety of roasted or stir-fried vegetables with your evening meal, this diversity of plant foods will give you exposure to what I have always called 'Nature's Edible Pharmacy'. We obviously know that plants are rich in vitamins and minerals, but they are also rich in powerful chemicals – called phytochemicals or phytonutrients. These can deliver almost drug-like effects in our body. They can reduce inflammation and pain. They can switch on key genes that help repair our cells and slow down ageing. They can support the immune system, support our eyesight, heal wounds more effectively and a thousand other benefits. Many of these compounds tend to be part of the chemistry that give plants their colour or their flavour, so the real key is diversity. Include as many plants with as many different colours and flavour profiles as possible to get maximum exposure to these substances.

### Up the three

This is a final little nugget that I feel is important for long-term good health. Fats are vitally important in our diet, and ensuring we get in a good amount of the right ones can safeguard us from some serious health issues down the line. The most important of these fats, from the point of view that most of us don't get anywhere near enough, is the omega-3 family of fatty acids – particularly EPA and DHA that we find in oily fish, algae (I know) and supplements.

These vital fats reduce inflammation in the body (a key driver of degenerative disease), help protect our arteries from damage, lower LDL cholesterol and increase levels of the 'good' HDL cholesterol, prevent brain shrinkage and neuronal damage, and support long-term cognitive function.

The best way to get more of these in is to include plenty of oily fish such as salmon, mackerel and herrings in your diet. If you follow a plant-based diet then you can get some DHA from algae such as spirulina, but to get the full spectrum of EPA and DHA you *must* use a supplement, which is very easy to come by.

These simple tips are not major lifestyle overhauls. They are not based on depriving yourself and following some silly rules that are impossible to stick to. You can still enjoy the food that you love and eat at your favourite restaurant, and easily support your long-term health. These simple tweaks to your day-to-day diet can help to protect you from the leading diet and lifestyle issues that plague our healthcare system: obesity, heart disease and type 2 diabetes, not to mention many preventable cancers. Why is that? Because these simple steps are doing the opposite to what our ultra-processed, highly refined diet is doing to our health. We know full well what these foods do. If we reverse-engineer that and build a lifestyle from doing the opposite, we give ourselves a fighting chance and have a sustainable plan of action that is easy to adopt for life.

In addition to Dale's advice above, there are some other simple ways to take back control:

## Regular exercise

Exercise can help regulate your hormones and boost your metabolism. Even moderate activities like walking or swimming can make a big difference. If walking seems unappealing, make the destination happy; meet a friend in the park. Dance to the radio around the house. Tidy the garden. Find some movement that brings you joy!

## Stress management

Stress can increase hunger and cravings. Practise stress-reducing activities like yoga, meditation or deep breathing exercises to help keep your hormones in check.

## Consistent sleep

Lack of sleep can disrupt your hormones and increase hunger. Aim for seven to eight hours of quality sleep each night to help regulate your appetite. Try to keep away from bright lights because they can hinder the production of melatonin, a hormone the body creates to help you sleep. There are tips on how to improve your sleep in Chapter 13.

Next, we're going to dive deep into a biological change that affects every woman at a certain time in her life.

## Case Study: How I Took Back Control

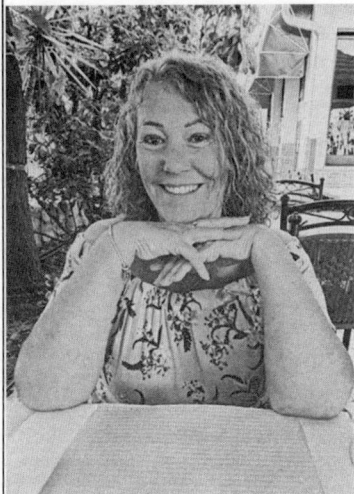

*Lorraine Murphy*

My claim to fame is that I stopped dieting and lost nearly 76kg (12st). Up to then, I felt like I was living in a fat suit – and I had no idea how to get out of it. I've been quite a big girl most of my life. Never mind obese, I used to call myself a beast!

I'd been dieting nearly all my life and I'd done them all – WeightWatchers, Slimming World, Atkins, Slimfast, something Sam Fox advertised years ago, the boiled egg diet, the cabbage soup diet, tablets from the doctor. After 44 years of dieting, none of them made a lasting difference.

I had a bad sugar addiction and I would think nothing of eating three chocolate bars a day. That's on top of cakes, biscuits, bread products, pastas. I knew the only way to end this habit was to break the sugar addiction, and so I kicked the elephant right out of the kitchen by doing the Slimpod programme.

I was a size 26, and I am now a size 16 bordering on 14, and I've lost 72.5kg (11st 6lb) without even thinking about it. Slimpod gave me my choices back. I could eat if I wanted to; if I didn't want to eat then fine.

Choosing healthy options just became natural and part of my life.

I'm now much more confident than I've ever been. I used to hate meeting people because I felt they were judging me because of my size. But now I'm the life and soul of the party – I'll go anywhere, meet anyone.

I feel like a normal person around food now. If there's cake or chocolate available, it's just automatic that I say no, but, actually, I don't say no every time. Sometimes I have a little treat. But I'm in control of the food rather than food being in control of me. I don't binge eat anymore at all.

I used to think nothing of having a bottle of wine in an evening. I would add crisps and peanuts, so I was just eating rubbish basically. The more sugar I consumed, the more I wanted. But it's completely stopped now. I'm in charge again.

*Find out more about Lorraine's story here:*

# CHAPTER 11

# Navigating the Menopause Minefield

For many women, the journey through perimenopause and then menopause can feel like an overwhelming whirlwind of changes, both physical and emotional. If you're noticing extra weight, particularly around your middle, despite your best efforts, then you're not alone and you're not doing anything wrong.

The changes you're experiencing are not because of a lack of willpower or a slower lifestyle, but are deeply rooted in the significant hormonal shifts happening in your body. These fluctuations have a direct impact on weight and fat distribution.

Menopause is a natural phase of life, but it doesn't have to be a time of struggle. By understanding the hormonal changes that occur and taking proactive steps to manage them, you can navigate menopause with greater ease and maintain a healthy weight. You have the power to take control of your health and make this stage of life one of empowerment and vitality.

One of the most notable changes in the run-up to and during menopause is the decline in oestrogen levels. Oestrogen is not just a reproductive hormone; it plays a crucial role in regulating metabolism, body fat distribution and even appetite. As oestrogen levels drop, the body compensates by storing more fat, particularly in the tummy area, where fat cells can produce a weaker form of oestrogen called oestrone. Unfortunately, oestrone is less effective than the oestrogen produced by the ovaries and is also more inflammatory, which can exacerbate weight gain and make it harder to lose excess fat.[1]

Other hormones, like ghrelin, leptin and cortisol, also start to behave differently. Ghrelin, the hunger hormone, tends to increase during menopause, leading to heightened feelings of hunger and stronger cravings.[2] Meanwhile, leptin, the hormone responsible for signalling when you're full, decreases, which means it takes longer for your brain to receive the message that you've had enough to eat.[3] This imbalance can lead to overeating, even when your calorie needs haven't changed.

Cortisol, the hormone released in response to stress, can also wreak havoc during menopause. With the various stresses that often go with this life stage – whether it's from physical symptoms like hot flushes or emotional stress from life's many demands – cortisol levels can rise. High cortisol levels not only contribute to fat storage, particularly around the abdomen, but also increase insulin resistance, making it harder for your body to manage blood sugar levels.[4]

The levels of dopamine (which, as we've seen, plays a key role in the brain's reward system) can fluctuate, which may lead to an increase in cravings for comfort foods. This is particularly challenging because these cravings often involve high-calorie, low-nutrient foods that can derail even the most disciplined eating plans.[5]

These hormonal changes don't just affect your appetite and fat storage; they also impact your metabolism. As oestrogen levels decline, there's a corresponding decrease in the body's ability to burn calories efficiently. This means that even if you're eating the same amount as you did before menopause, you might still gain weight.[6]

Additionally, the loss of muscle mass, which naturally occurs as we age, further slows down our metabolism. Since muscle burns more calories than fat, less muscle means fewer calories burned at rest, contributing to gradual weight gain over time.

Sleep disturbances, which are common during menopause, can further complicate weight management. Oestrogen plays a role in regulating sleep, so, when levels drop, sleep patterns can be disrupted. Hot flushes and night sweats are common culprits, but changes in the sleep hormone melatonin and increased cortisol levels can also lead to poor sleep.[7] When you don't get enough rest, it affects the balance of leptin and ghrelin, making you more likely to overeat and crave high-calorie foods.[8]

The good news is that, while these changes are challenging, they're not insurmountable. By understanding the science behind menopausal weight gain, you can take targeted action to manage your weight and improve your overall well-being.

It's also worth mentioning the role of hormone replacement therapy (HRT). While HRT is not suitable for everyone, it can be an effective way to manage some of the symptoms of menopause, including weight gain. Research has shown that HRT can help reduce the accumulation of visceral fat (the dangerous fat around your organs), lower blood glucose and insulin levels, and even positively influence gut health.[9] If you're considering HRT, it's important to discuss it with your doctor to weigh up the benefits and risks based on your individual health profile.

Finally, it's important to approach weight management during menopause with a sense of self-compassion and patience. This is a time of significant change, and it's normal to feel frustrated or overwhelmed. However, by taking small, consistent steps towards better health – whether that's improving your diet, moving more or managing stress – you can regain control and feel more confident in your body. Remember, it's not about perfection; it's about progress.

## How You Can Take Back Control
### Eat more plants
Try eating the Mediterranean way (there's more about this on page 224). Include foods like flaxseeds, soya and legumes in your daily diet to help naturally balance oestrogen levels. Studies have indicated that these plant-based foods can mimic the effects of oestrogen, providing some people with relief from menopausal symptoms.[10]

### Get physical regularly
Engage in regular exercise to boost metabolism, manage stress and improve mood. Strength training is particularly effective for maintaining muscle mass and supporting metabolic health. The NHS recommends at least 150 minutes of moderate exercise or 75 minutes of vigorous exercise a week.

*Be a mindful eater*

Pay attention to hunger and fullness cues to avoid over-eating. Drink plenty of water, as thirst can sometimes be mistaken for hunger. Practising mindful eating – being aware of why and what you eat – helps you develop a healthier relationship with food.

*Get enough sleep*

Ensure you get sufficient sleep to help regulate the hormones that affect appetite and stress levels. Good sleep is essential and I deal with this in depth in Chapter 13.

*Reduce stress*

Build meditation, deep breathing or yoga into your daily routine to manage stress effectively. Find time to relax, and time to be yourself.

In the next chapter, you'll discover a lot more about how the stress hormone affects the size of your waistline and what you can do about it.

# Case Study: How I Took Back Control

*Rachael Buckett*

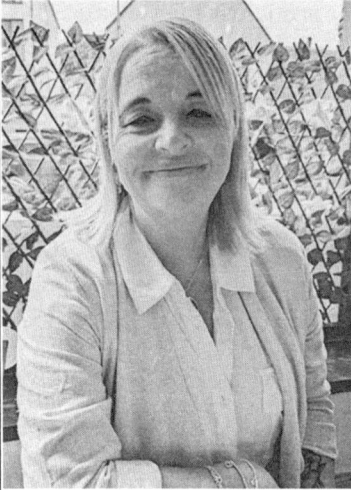

Two years ago, I was at my lowest point. I was 120.5kg (19st), a size 24, struggling to move and seriously considering drastic measures like gastric surgery. I felt utterly out of control with my weight and health.

I was coming up to 50, with the menopause fast approaching, and thought 'this must be what an 80-year-old feels like.' I started researching online and stumbled upon Slimpod, which promised a different approach to weight loss.

Within two years, I was 44kg (7st) lighter, and the transformation was astonishing. The best part wasn't just the weight loss, but how my mindset shifted from day one. I finally believed that I could take control of my health, and I was determined to do whatever it took. It wasn't about dieting anymore. It was about changing my habits and putting myself first. Everything went brilliantly – I was in control of my weight.

Then, suddenly, the menopause kicked in and the problems started in my head. I'd always been told the menopause meant it was impossible to lose weight and that its onset meant you lost control. Today, I know that's untrue, but the voice in my head told me all my success was doomed to fail and that I would fall off the wagon. And I did!

I went to pieces, my healthy mindset changed and, before I knew it, I had put almost 13kg (30lb) back on. I spoke to Sandra and she advised me to go back to doing what I had loved most before the menopause – exercise. Exercise had become a natural part of my life, which I never thought I'd say. I work from home, so since I'd been on Slimpod, I'd started the day with a dog walk and added in 30 minutes of running. At lunchtime, I walked the dog again, and most days I hit 10,000 steps before my afternoon even began. After work, I either went for a bike ride or another long walk. Some days I did both! My daily step count had consistently been over 13,000 for the previous six months.

My self-limiting belief about the menopause stopped all that in its tracks. So I told myself I had to get a grip and start working my body again. It wasn't easy at first, but, once my positive mindset kicked in again, things started to happen.

Slimpod has helped me make big changes in my lifestyle. I no longer use the car for short trips, preferring to walk or cycle. Not only does it keep me active, but it's less stressful, better for the environment and saves money on petrol. I've cut down on TV too, watching no more than an hour a day. It's amazing how much more time I have now for things that matter.

Food-wise, I eat when I'm hungry and focus on

whole, nutritious foods. I drink more water, and though I allow myself some coffee and the occasional glass of wine, sugary treats are no longer a daily habit. I haven't cut out 'bad' foods entirely, but I've learned to enjoy them in moderation.

The difference in my life is staggering. I've dropped from a size 24 to a size 10, 12 or 14, depending on the shop. I feel more confident, happier and healthier than I ever have. I don't hide behind oversized, dark clothes anymore – I actually enjoy shopping for bright, colourful outfits. Even my husband has noticed the change. He says I'm more confident and stand up for myself more, which is true. I'm no longer invisible, and I know my opinion matters.

I'm never going back to that old life, and I'm excited for what the future holds.

*Find out more about Rachael's story here:*

## CHAPTER 12

# How Stress Increases Tummy Fat

The key to achieving a healthy body isn't just the food you eat or the exercise you do; it's also in the calm moments you carve out for yourself amid the chaos of life. Stress, an inevitable part of life, can have a profound impact on your body's ability to manage weight.

So we're going to explore how stress affects your hormones and why managing stress is crucial for sustainable weight loss and well-being.

We all recognise the comforting attraction of a bar of chocolate or the sweet allure of a doughnut when stress levels soar. These aren't just cravings; they're signals from our body that it's seeking a brief respite from stress. Emotional eating becomes a way of coping, a momentary fix that soon leads to guilt and a cycle of stress and overeating. There's a whole chapter on that coming up later.

Stress profoundly influences our eating patterns. Scientific research reveals that stress triggers the release of hormones like adrenaline and cortisol.[1] Adrenaline is the immediate response, getting our heart racing and ready for action. Cortisol, on the other hand, lingers, and when stress becomes chronic, cortisol convinces our bodies to store fat, particularly around the waist, increasing the risk of various health problems.[2]

The mix of adrenaline and cortisol can lead to immediate disruptions and long-term health declines, such as lower bone density and higher blood sugar levels. Research indicates that stress-induced cortisol secretion is also consistently greater among women with tummy fat, highlighting the connection between stress and abdominal weight gain. Similarly, a study found that stress slows metabolism and increases the likelihood of fat storage, particularly in response to high-fat, high-sugar foods.[3]

Stress doesn't just impact our hormones; it also affects our nutrient levels. It demands high-energy performances from our bodies, depleting vitamins C and B, as well as minerals like magnesium and zinc.[4] Moreover, stress often leads us to crave high-sugar, high-fat foods, further depleting these vital nutrients and creating a vicious cycle.[5]

So, how do we manage stress effectively to restore balance? It starts with creating daily moments of relaxation and finding personal sanctuaries amid life's hustle. One approach to finding this balance is mindfulness, proven to reduce stress and improve emotional regulation.[6]

Regular physical activity is another key strategy to tune our mood and keep stress at bay. Research shows that exercise acts as a buffer against stress, enhancing psychological resilience and reducing cortisol levels.[7] You don't have to run a marathon to make a difference; brisk walks at least three times a week can be hugely beneficial.

Adequate sleep is also vital. Quality sleep helps regulate hormones that affect appetite and stress levels, while research shows that sleep deprivation negatively impacts the regulation of hunger hormones, increasing the risk of weight gain.[8] Establishing a regular sleep schedule, creating a restful environment and practising relaxation techniques before bed can improve sleep quality and support overall health. Sleep is so important that there's a whole chapter on it coming up next.

Understanding the complex interplay between hormones, brain function and behaviour under stress allows you to tailor your approach to health. By focusing on strategies that support hormonal balance and overall well-being – such as those outlined overleaf – you can turn this challenging phase into an opportunity for health empowerment.

## How You Can Take Back Control

*Daily relaxation*

The mind is a powerful organ, controlling up to 90 per cent of our actions and reactions. It's the unconscious part that manages our breathing, our heartbeat and even our immune system. However, despite its huge strength, it's also susceptible to the negative impacts of stress. Engage in activities that quieten the mind, such as meditation or deep breathing exercises.

*Regular exercise*

Find joy in physical activities that boost endorphins, one of nature's pleasure hormones, and improve your mood.

*Create a support team*

Surround yourself with friends who uplift and support you, and avoid those who drain you – I call them psychic vampires, because they suck the energy out of you.

*Eat more nutrients*

Consume a balanced diet rich in vitamins and minerals to counteract the depletion caused by stress (see page 88).

*Build resilience*

Develop coping strategies to handle stress gracefully. Take several deep breaths, close your eyes and count to ten until the internal pressure subsides. Try to bounce back and learn from adversity.

## Case Study: How I Took Back Control

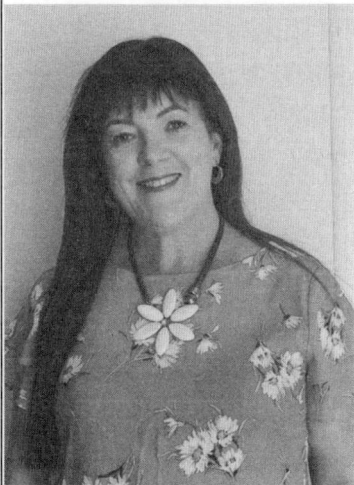

*Biddy O'Sullivan*

For years, anxiety and stress ruled my life. I was often too afraid to leave the house, trapped in an emotionally abusive relationship, and had become a shadow of my former self.

The turning point came 20 years ago when I had a severe panic attack at a Madonna concert. Since then, I'd been living a half-life, avoiding anything that might trigger another attack. I stopped going to gigs, theatres and even the cinema. The anxiety was so severe that I once stood outside a supermarket, too terrified to go in because what I needed was at the back of the shop. The thought of having a panic attack far from the exit was paralysing.

But things changed dramatically when I discovered a new approach to managing my well-being. Slimpod wasn't just about losing weight; it was about reclaiming my life. Over the past year, I've done more than I have in the last two decades.

I hadn't been on an airplane for 13 years, but I started small with a flight from Dublin to Kerry. From there, I gained the confidence to travel more – first to Edinburgh, then to Mallorca, Paris and even Disneyland. It's incredible how freeing it feels to no longer be held back by fear.

In the past year alone, I've gone on four holidays, attended numerous concerts and started a new job. Just last night, I went to an indoor Liam Gallagher concert. It was a huge moment for me. I was a little nervous, but, for the first time in 12 years, I wasn't constantly checking the exits. The stadium was packed, but I stayed calm and enjoyed the show. That's a massive win for me – something I never thought I could do again.

Although I still face challenges, the difference now is that I don't give up. Even when it's scary, I keep going. I've also noticed that my new-found confidence is spilling over into other areas of my life. I'm more confident at work, I exercise daily and, for the first time in a long time, I like what I see when I look in the mirror.

My approach to eating has changed too. I used to comfort eat, grabbing a biscuit or two in the mornings to soothe my anxiety. I ate without thinking, just because it was time to eat. Now, I eat when I'm hungry and stop when I'm full. It's a simple shift, but it's been life-changing. My cravings are gone, and I'm finally in tune with my body's needs.

More importantly, I've regained my joy and confidence. I'm finally living my life on my terms, and it feels amazing.

*Find out more about Biddy's story here:*

# CHAPTER 13

# Poor Sleep Sabotages Weight Loss

Here's a fact that might surprise you: if you have fewer than 7 hours of sleep for 14 nights in a row, you go into fat storage mode and keep 50 per cent of the fat you would have released if you'd been sleeping longer.[1]

Imagine trying to navigate your day on a half-charged battery. That's essentially what you do to your body when you skimp on sleep. Sleep is the time when your body repairs itself, rebalances its chemicals and processes the day's activities.[2]

With the understanding that sleep is not just a passive state but an active, integral component of health, including weight loss, we can begin to treat it with the attention it deserves; not just for better nights, but also for better days, filled with energy and vitality.

There are four main ways in which poor sleep can sabotage your weight-loss efforts, primarily through its complex interactions with hormones and metabolism. Let's break it down:

## It increases blood sugar levels

When you don't get enough sleep, your body's ability to handle blood sugar can go haywire. After just four nights of poor sleep, you can become insulin resistant. Insulin is a hormone that helps control your blood sugar levels. When it doesn't work properly, your body starts storing more fat. One study found that after a few nights of bad sleep, insulin sensitivity dropped by over 30 per cent.[3] This means your body is more likely to hold on to fat, making weight loss harder.

## It leads to hormone imbalance

Sleep also plays a crucial role in maintaining a healthy balance of the hormones ghrelin and leptin (see page 80). When you're sleep-deprived, your body produces more ghrelin and less leptin.[4] This imbalance makes you feel hungrier and less satisfied after meals, often leading to overeating. Plus, research shows that when you're tired, you're more likely to reach for unhealthy food.[5]

## It affects your metabolism

A striking illustration of the importance of sleep comes from research suggesting that with fewer than seven hours of sleep over two weeks, the amount of fat lost can be cut in half compared to those who sleep more.[6] This is because without adequate sleep, your metabolism slows, and your body holds on to fat more tenaciously.

## It reduces self-control

Ever noticed how a poor night's sleep makes that doughnut at work look even more irresistible? That's not just a feeling; it's an actual physiological response. Lack of sleep diminishes your self-control and decision-making abilities, making it harder to make healthy choices. So it's not so much that if you sleep more you'll lose fat, but if you have too little sleep, it messes up your metabolism and contributes to weight gain.

Recognising sleep as a pillar of weight loss empowers you to take control from another angle. Your well-being is not just about diet and exercise; it's about giving your body the rest it needs to function at its best. It's about seeing sleep not just as downtime but as a critical component of a healthy life-style. By improving sleep, you enhance your body's natural abilities to regulate appetite and metabolism, making your weight-loss journey smoother and more sustainable. And who knows? You might just find yourself feeling more ener-gised and less tempted by those sneaky late-night snacks.

## How You Can Take Back Control
### Establish a routine
Routine is king, so stick to a sleep schedule. Consistency is key in signalling to your body when it's time to wind down. Go to bed and wake up at the same time every day, even on weekends, to reinforce your body's sleep–wake cycle. Aim for at least seven to eight hours' sleep a night.

### Create a restful space
Optimise your space by ensuring your sleeping environ-ment is cool, quiet and dark. Invest in good-quality bedding and consider blackout curtains or a white noise machine if needed.

Engage in relaxing pre-sleep rituals such as reading a book or taking a warm bath. Consider using apps that guide you through relaxing meditations or provide ambient sounds to help you sleep. A vital part of my Slimpod programme is the Chillpod relaxation audio, which people swear by.

## No late eating or drinking

Avoid heavy meals and vigorous exercise in the three hours or so before bedtime. Both can disrupt your ability to fall asleep, as can nicotine, caffeine and alcohol. Incorporate relaxation practices like yoga or meditation in your evening routine instead to help prepare your mind and body for sleep.

## Hide away the phone

Exposure to blue light from phone screens and tablets can disrupt your natural sleep cycle by suppressing the body's release of melatonin, a hormone that makes us feel drowsy.[7] If you must use devices, use night shift settings that reduce blue light exposure in the evening.

# PART THREE

# Reverse, Reset and Retrain: Your Role in Your Change

This is where you become empowered to fight back and take control. In this part, discover the modern advances in neuroscience that mean you're no longer a slave to your brain, but can retrain it to have a whole new relationship with food.

## CHAPTER 14

# Drive a Wedge Into Emotional Eating

Over the years I've been running my Slimpod programme, it's become obvious that one of the main reasons people struggle to sustain long-term weight loss is emotional eating.

My Diet Dossier survey of people who had spent years dieting before joining Slimpod revealed that 96.8 per cent identified as comfort eaters or full-on emotional eaters. The top three triggers? Boredom, stress and tiredness.

Emotional eating is defined as 'the practice of consuming food in response to an emotional trigger'.[1] When emotions take control, food becomes a coping mechanism, a way to fill a void or a reward. Amazingly, it's rarely apples, celery or carrots that we turn to, but more often biscuits, cake, crisps or even alcohol – and sometimes all of these. The foods of choice are often refined carbohydrates and sweets providing temporary relief but leading to long-term issues with weight and health.[2]

This behaviour can start at a very young age. Parents, often emotionally and physically unavailable, might give their children sweet foods to keep them occupied when they're busy.

Consequently, children begin to associate food with love and comfort. When they feel unhappy or stressed, they turn to food, especially sugary or comforting foods, as a coping mechanism.[3] This habit can persist into adulthood, making emotional eating a significant challenge.

I know that my love of chocolate started when I was at school. My parents owned a grocery shop and were very busy seven days a week. To reward me for doing my homework after school, I was allowed to choose a chocolate from the shop. This daily treat created an association in my brain: chocolate equalled pleasure. This association became dangerous because whenever I was unhappy, I would reach for chocolate to feel better. And, of course, it worked, albeit temporarily.

## Is Food Giving You a Hug?

The challenge with emotional eating is that many people don't realise they're doing it. In my weekly Zoom sessions and live chats, I often bring up the topic with those who are struggling. Many haven't considered themselves emotional eaters, saying they eat when they're bored. But boredom eating is a form of emotional eating, just as much as reaching for food for comfort or reward.

If you find yourself turning to comfort foods and binge eating when stressed, bored, sad or lonely, you may be an emotional eater.[4] You might snack at your desk to deal with work stresses, even when you're not hungry.

Awareness is the first step. Once you acknowledge the behaviour, the big question becomes: how do you stop? First, you need to understand the emotional triggers. What is the food providing? Comfort from stress or sadness, or relief from boredom? Has food become a friend because of loneliness? Or is it a reward for a hard day?

Sometimes, food reflects how we feel about ourselves. Low self-esteem can drive us to seek solace in eating.[5] Ask yourself, is food giving you a hug? Then, delve deeper. What emotional comfort do you get from that food?

This awareness brings subconscious actions to the conscious mind, enabling you to make choices. Food should be fuel, not laden with emotional meanings. Understanding these feelings disrupts automatic patterns and brings them to your conscious attention.

It's also vitally important to be able to identify the two different kinds of hunger:

1. Emotional hunger is urgent – a need that feels immediate and out of control, hijacking your mind. It often involves cravings for specific foods, leading to mindless and rapid eating, especially of ultra-processed carbs and sugary foods. This need overrides common sense and can lead to feelings of guilt and shame.[6]
2. Real hunger comes on gradually, led by physical signals like a rumbling stomach and a sense of emptiness and low fuel. You remain in control, eating when ready, allowing time to make healthy choices. Real hunger means your mind–body communication is working perfectly, unlike emotional hunger where stress, tiredness and the need for comfort dominate.[7]

Another way to stop emotional eating is to drive a wedge in the subconscious behaviour that's causing it. This empowers you to think rationally about what you're doing instead of automated behaviour running your life. Then you have the choice about whether or not to eat that cake or drink that glass of wine. Once you make that rational decision, it's the beginning of the end of you being at the mercy of food and drink.

The following technique is a really good way of creating some distance from the urge or craving. Have a go because it works![8]

## Cost benefit analysis

Cost benefit analysis, or CBA for short, helps you weigh up the pros and cons of your behaviour so you can make more informed decisions. When you create the distance between yourself and the thought/feeling/image of food, it's easier to tell yourself: 'There's no comfort in food. Food is fuel and that's it. Food is never going to be a long-term comfort blanket – it just makes me unhappy.' CBA can be a powerful tool to understand why you turn to food for comfort (or many other reasons) and how you can develop healthier coping mechanisms.

Here's how CBA works. Divide a sheet of paper into two columns: one for the costs and one for the benefits. Then write down the short- and long-term benefits and costs of emotional eating.

There are two main short-term benefits:

1. **Temporary relief:** Eating can provide instant gratification or immediate comfort and distraction from an emotional

trigger or upset. It reduces the negative emotions by providing a pleasurable experience.[9]

2. **Taste satisfaction:** The sensory pleasure of eating, especially comfort foods high in sugar and fat, can enhance mood momentarily. This is because of the release of dopamine (see page 16).[10]

Consider if either of these particularly applies to you and write down a few bullet point details.

Two of the immediate costs of emotional eating are guilt and shame, especially if the emotional eating conflicts with your health goals or weight-loss efforts. This negative emotional response can make the initial emotional trigger stronger, creating a vicious cycle.

When it comes to the long-term benefits of emotional eating, there aren't any! The temporary pleasure does not address the underlying emotional issues and almost always leads to negative consequences.

The long-term costs are worrying. The first is weight gain and health issues; consistently turning to food for emotional relief will make you put on weight and increase the risk of health problems such as diabetes and heart disease.[11]

The other sad cost is emotional dependence. Relying on food to manage your feelings can prevent you from developing healthier coping mechanisms. By eating you're not dealing with the problem, you're merely pushing it under the carpet.

Embrace these strategies with compassion and persistence, and watch as you transform your eating habits and emotional well-being. Overcoming emotional eating isn't just about changing your eating habits; it's about holistic self-care. Embrace self-love and compassion, recognising that you deserve to feel good without relying on food for comfort. Believe in your ability to make lasting changes and take it one step at a time. Each step towards healthier coping mechanisms is a step towards a happier, more balanced life.

One word of caution: emotional roots of eating habits can be deep and associated with trauma or other significant events, often in childhood.[12] For some people, one-to-one therapy with a professional can be invaluable. Therapy helps you to understand and address underlying issues, guiding healthier coping strategies for long-term recovery.

## How You Can Take Back Control

### Acknowledge you do it

Awareness is the first step to changing the habit. Recognise that you use food to feel better. Understanding the root cause helps develop healthier coping mechanisms.

### Recognise the triggers

Keep a journal to track situations and emotions that trigger emotional eating. Identify what drives you to eat emotionally. Is it stress, boredom or sadness? Understanding your triggers helps you prepare for and manage them better – and if you know your triggers are coming, you can then address them directly before they take hold, so there's no urge to turn to food.

## Be a mindful eater

Be present while eating. Think about your food and enjoy the flavours, textures and experience of your meal. This helps break the cycle of mindless, emotional eating.

## Find new comforts

Discover other sources of comfort and joy. Make a list of healthier ways to cope with emotions, such as exercise, meditation, reading a good book or talking to a friend. These activities can replace the need for food as an emotional crutch and give you alternatives you can quickly turn to when you feel the urge to eat emotionally.

## Treat yourself with care

Offer yourself the right self-care and kindness, much like you would a young child. Don't write yourself off as worthless or a failure just because you had a piece of chocolate or three crisps. You're just being human.

## List the costs and benefits

Be brutally honest with yourself about the temporary pleasure versus the lasting consequences. Seeing these factors on paper can provide clarity and motivation for change.

## Review and reflect

Regularly review your CBA list and reflect on your progress. Adjust your strategies as needed and celebrate small victories. This helps reinforce positive changes and keeps you motivated.

# Case Study: How I Took Back Control

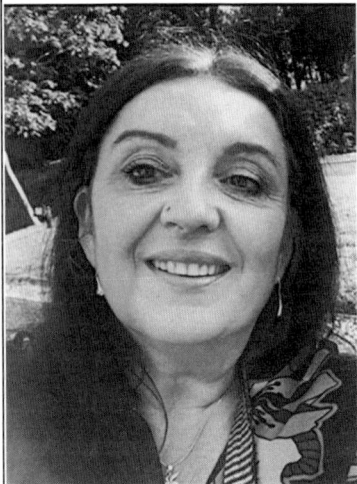

*Michelle Marshall*

I grew up believing that my weight defined me. My first diet was at 15, driven by constant comparisons to my grandmother, who was a large woman. I heard time and again, 'Be careful, or you'll end up like your grandma.' And, sure enough, that label became my reality.

It's amazing how easily we live up to the labels given to us, even unintentionally. For much of my life, my achievements were overshadowed by how much I weighed. Despite excelling academically and in other areas, it felt like none of it mattered if I wasn't slim.

Over the years, I've tried countless diets and exercise plans. I'd push myself to the limit, but it was never sustainable. Then I discovered a different approach with Slimpod, and everything changed. My journey hasn't been quick or drastic, but it's been transformative. Though I'm still carrying some extra weight, I'm no longer classified as clinically obese. That alone feels like an enormous victory. Now, I walk my dog daily, often for two hours, but I never do less than forty-five minutes.

I've stopped panicking about food. If I want to eat out, I do. I no longer feel like I'm putting my life on hold. I'm getting better at eating when I'm actually hungry, rather than eating out of stress or habit. It's no longer about being thin for others; it's about feeling good in my own skin.

My husband loves me as I am, and I've come to accept and love myself too. The confidence that comes with this acceptance is incredible. I no longer put off living. I don't say, 'I'll do that when I lose weight'; I do everything now – belly dancing included! The belly dancing community is amazing – so supportive and body-positive. I never feel self-conscious there, and I don't let anything hold me back anymore.

I've gone from a size 22 to a size 16 or 18. My bra size has changed, and my stamina has increased significantly. I still have some weight to lose, and I'm not done yet. But I feel better in my clothes, I'm fitter and I'm healthier. I'm also so much happier and more confident. Every day, I'm learning and making progress. My journey isn't over, but I'm loving the direction it's taking. Life is too short to wait for an arbitrary number on the scale.

*Find out more about Michelle's story here:*

## CHAPTER 15

# Escape From a Mental Groove

We've all been there: you start a new diet or fitness plan, full of hope and determination, but, before long, you find yourself back in old habits, feeling defeated and wondering where it all went wrong. If this sounds familiar, you're not alone, and the explanation goes deeper than just willpower. What you've experienced is likely because of something known as cognitive loops.

Cognitive loops are powerful cycles of thought and behaviour that can trap you in unhelpful patterns, making it difficult to achieve your weight-loss goals. They are essentially feedback circuits in your brain where your thoughts, feelings and actions reinforce one another, creating a cycle that's hard to break. Think of it like an old vinyl record stuck in a groove, playing the same track over and over again. But instead of music, it's a loop of self-doubt, negative thinking or behaviours that don't serve your best interests. These loops can make it feel like you're constantly struggling against yourself, and they can be incredibly frustrating.

The science behind cognitive loops is both fascinating and empowering. At the core of this concept is neuroplasticity, which is the brain's ability to reorganise itself by forming new neural connections throughout life.[1] Your brain is always changing, shaped by your experiences, thoughts and actions. However, this can work both for and against you. When you repeatedly think about or do something, your brain strengthens the neural pathways associated with that behaviour, making it more automatic over time. This is why certain patterns of thinking or behaviour can feel so deeply entrenched – it's as if your brain has hardwired itself to keep repeating them.

Consider how this plays out in the context of weight loss. Imagine you've just started a diet, and things are going well initially. But then, something happens – you have a stressful day at work, you miss a workout or you indulge in a slice of cake. This triggers a cascade of negative thoughts: 'I've ruined everything' or 'I'll never succeed.' These thoughts lead to feelings of guilt and frustration, which might cause you to abandon your healthy habits altogether.

This is a classic cognitive loop: trigger, behaviour and reinforcement. The more often you go through this loop, the stronger it becomes, making it more likely that you'll repeat the same pattern in the future.

Research has shown that these loops can be particularly powerful when it comes to food and eating habits. For instance, studies on the brain's reward system reveal that when you consume high-calorie foods, your brain releases dopamine.[2] As we've seen, this dopamine hit creates a reward loop, where you start to crave those foods more and more, even when you know they're not in line with your health goals. Over time, this loop can become so powerful that it overrides your conscious intentions to eat healthily.

But cognitive loops aren't just about what you eat – they also involve how you think. Take, for example, the moment you step on the scales and see a number you didn't want to see. That number can trigger a loop of negative thoughts: 'I'm never going to lose weight' or 'What's the point in trying?' These thoughts can lead to behaviours like comfort eating or skipping exercise, which reinforce the belief that you can't succeed. And so the cycle continues.

The good news is that while cognitive loops are powerful, they're not unbreakable. Understanding how they work is the first step towards disrupting them.

Because of neuroplasticity, the same brain mechanism that created these loops can also be used to break them. By intervening in the loop – changing the trigger, the behaviour or the reinforcement – you can weaken the loop over time and replace it with new, more positive patterns. For example, if you find that you often reach for unhealthy foods when you're stressed, the first step is to recognise that stress is your trigger. Once you've identified the trigger, you can work on changing your response.

Instead of turning to food, you might try a different behaviour, like taking a few deep breaths, going for a short walk or practising mindfulness. These alternative behaviours can help you manage your stress without resorting to food, and over time your brain will start to form new neural connections that support these healthier habits.

One of the most effective strategies for disrupting cognitive loops is cognitive restructuring. This technique involves recognising and challenging the negative thoughts that drive the loop. For instance, instead of thinking, 'I've failed because

I ate that slice of cake', you could reframe the thought as 'I enjoyed a treat but that doesn't mean I've failed. I can make a healthier choice next time.' By consciously changing your thoughts, you can break the loop and prevent it from triggering the same negative behaviours.

Another powerful approach is to focus on making small, consistent changes rather than trying to overhaul your entire lifestyle at once. Research suggests that small, manageable changes are more sustainable and less likely to trigger cognitive loops of failure.[3] For instance, instead of setting a goal to lose a significant amount of weight quickly, you might focus on eating one more serving of vegetables each day or walking for an extra ten minutes. These small victories can create positive reinforcement, gradually weakening the old, negative loops and replacing them with new, healthier ones.

It's also crucial to address the emotional aspect of cognitive loops. Feelings of failure, guilt and shame can be incredibly powerful, but they don't have to define your journey. Practising self-compassion – treating yourself with the same kindness you would offer a friend – can help reduce the emotional charge that reinforces the loop.[4] Instead of beating yourself up after a slip-up, try to approach it with curiosity rather than judgement. Ask yourself what led to the slip-up, what you can learn from it and how you can approach things differently next time.

What's truly empowering about breaking cognitive loops is the realisation that you have the power to change your brain. It's not easy, and it won't happen overnight, but with patience and persistence, you can rewire your brain for success. Each time you interrupt a cognitive loop, you're taking a step towards creating new neural pathways that support your goals. Over time, these new pathways will become stronger, and the old, unhelpful loops will weaken and eventually fade.

It's also important to remember that cognitive loops don't just affect weight loss – they can impact many areas of your life, from your relationships to your work. By learning to recognise and disrupt these loops, you're not just improving your chances of losing weight, you're also developing a valuable skill that can enhance your overall well-being.

So, if you find yourself stuck in a cycle of self-defeating thoughts or behaviours, remember that change is possible. The fact that your brain is capable of forming cognitive loops means it's also capable of breaking them. With the right strategies, you can disrupt the patterns that are holding you back and create new, positive loops that propel you towards your goals.

Understanding the science behind cognitive loops gives you the tools to take back control. Rather than feeling trapped by old patterns, you can approach your weight-loss journey with a sense of empowerment and possibility. You're not at the mercy of your brain – you're in the driver's seat and, with each step, you're steering towards a healthier, happier you.

## How You Can Take Back Control

*Identify your triggers*

Start by recognising what triggers your cognitive loops. Whether it's stress, boredom or specific situations, being aware of the trigger allows you to intervene early. When you notice a trigger, pause and choose a different response.

*Reframe negative thoughts*

Challenge the negative thoughts that reinforce your cognitive loops. Instead of focusing on failure, reframe your thoughts to focus on what you can do differently next time. This shift in perspective can weaken the loop and promote more positive behaviours.

*Live a positive life*

Find activities that bring you joy and satisfaction that don't involve food. Hobbies, physical activities or social events can help take your mind off food and reduce the likelihood of emotional eating.

*Focus on small wins*

Break the cycle of all-or-nothing thinking by celebrating small victories. Each positive change, no matter how minor, can help create new, positive cognitive loops that support your long-term goals.

In the next chapter, we'll look at six ways your brain distorts your thoughts in a negative way and how you can push back and be positive.

# Case Study: How I Took Back Control

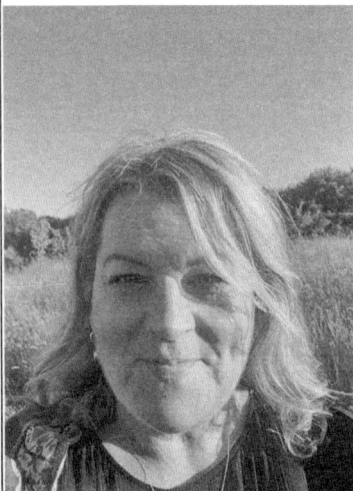

*Charlotte Donovan*

I've been overweight since I was 15, so that's 40 years of not believing I'd ever be slim. I was always the bigger girl, the one who stood out for all the wrong reasons. My relationship with food was deeply tied to my childhood, which was fraught with emotional turmoil.

Growing up in a difficult household, I turned to sugar for comfort. It was the one thing that soothed me when everything else felt chaotic. But what started as a coping mechanism quickly spiralled into a lifelong habit.

By my thirties, I was diagnosed with polycystic ovary syndrome, a condition that made it even harder to manage my weight. Then, in my late forties, I was told I had prediabetes. By the time I hit my fifties, I was officially diagnosed with type 2 diabetes. It was terrifying, but instead of taking action, I felt paralysed.

I was stuck in a cycle of denial, frustration and fear. Whenever a doctor would tell me to 'eat less and move more', it only added to my sense of hopelessness. I knew what I needed to do, but I couldn't seem to do it. I was trapped in a cycle of yo-yo dieting, losing and regaining the same 20kg (3st) over and over again.

For years, I felt out of control, as if my body was a

burden I had to carry. I had no idea how to break free from the habits that had been ingrained in me for so long. I felt like a prisoner to my cravings, especially for sugar. Every time I tried to cut back, I'd end up back where I started, or worse.

But a few months ago, I discovered Slimpod, a new approach that didn't focus on dieting but on mindset. I began making healthier choices without any pressure and I began eating more mindfully, choosing nutritious foods because they made me feel good, not because I had to. I also joined a gym and, for the first time, began to enjoy exercising. My whole mindset had changed from punishing my body to nurturing it. Over the next six months, I gradually lost about 6kg (1st) and dropped a dress size.

The most remarkable change, however, was my health. My doctor confirmed that I was no longer diabetic – not even prediabetic. I've lost a dress size, but, more importantly, I've gained control over my life. The desire for sugar that once ruled me has faded. I find myself genuinely craving healthy foods, and the idea of 'falling off the wagon' doesn't apply anymore because I was never on one to begin with.

This journey has been about so much more than weight loss. It's been about reclaiming my life and discovering the person I was meant to be. I can't wait to see where this new-found confidence takes me next.

*Find out more about Charlotte's story here:*

## CHAPTER 16

# Challenge Your Distorted Thoughts About Food

My best-attended Facebook Live chats are when I discuss the distorted thoughts we have, leading us down a path of self-doubt and self-sabotage.

In psychology, distorted thoughts are known as cognitive distortions.[1] These are irrational and often harmful thought patterns that really interfere with progress and success, and this can be in anything you do, not just weight loss. They influence your emotions and your behaviour. They are beliefs that limit your ability to reach your goals and dreams. These mental filters skew our perception of reality, leading us to make inaccurate and often negative interpretations of our experiences.

When it comes to our relationship with food, cognitive distortions can play a major role, often exacerbating issues such as emotional eating, binge eating and negative body image. Understanding these distortions and learning how to challenge them is crucial for developing a healthier relationship with food.

There are six common cognitive distortions:

## All-or-nothing thinking

This distortion, also known as black-and-white thinking, involves viewing situations in extreme black-and-white terms. For example, you might think: 'I ate a slice of cake, so I've ruined my diet completely.' This mindset can cause a cycle of strict dieting followed by binge eating, as any deviation from perfection is seen as a total failure.[2]

## Over-generalisation

This is when you draw broad, negative conclusions based on a single event. If you have one setback, such as overeating at a party, you might conclude: 'I'll never be able to control my eating habits.' This type of thinking can demotivate you and make it difficult to maintain healthy eating behaviours.[3]

## Catastrophising

This is the tendency to expect the worst possible outcome from a situation. You might think: 'If I don't stick to my diet perfectly, I'll gain a lot of weight and be unhealthy.' This fear can create unnecessary anxiety around food and eating, leading to stress and potentially unhealthy eating patterns.[4]

## Labelling

Labelling involves assigning a fixed, negative label to yourself based on specific behaviours. For example, after overeating you might label yourself as 'a failure' or 'hopeless'. This negative self-perception can erode your self-esteem and make it challenging to adopt a balanced, healthy relationship with food.[5]

## Mind-reading

This occurs when you assume you know what others think about you.[6] You might believe they are judging you harshly for your eating habits or body size, even when there is no evidence to support this. This can lead to social anxiety and further emotional eating as a way to cope with the perceived judgement.

## Emotional reasoning

This is when you believe that because you feel a certain way, it must be true. For instance, if you feel guilty after eating a dessert, you might conclude that eating dessert is inherently bad. This can lead to unhealthy restrictive eating patterns.[7]

The first important step in challenging cognitive distortions is to become aware of them.[8] Pay attention to your thoughts around food and eating, and notice when they fall into the six patterns set out above.

Once you've identified a distorted thought, you must question its validity. Ask yourself if there is evidence to support this thought or if you might be exaggerating.[9] For example, if you think, 'I've ruined my diet by eating this cake', challenge that and reduce its impact by considering the bigger picture of your overall eating habits and goals.

Reframe your thinking by replacing distorted thoughts with more balanced, rational ones. Instead of thinking: 'I'm a failure for eating this dessert', reframe it to: 'I enjoyed a dessert, and that's okay. One indulgence doesn't define my overall eating habits.' This shift in perspective can help reduce negative emotions.

Self-compassion is vital. Be kind to yourself and recognise that everyone has setbacks. Treat yourself with the same understanding and kindness that you would offer to a friend. This can help you become resilient and move past slip-ups without falling into a cycle of guilt and shame.[10]

## How You Can Take Back Control

*Eat mindfully*

Pay full attention to your food and the experience of eating. This involves noticing the colours, smells, textures and flavours of your food. Being present, conscious and engaged when you're eating can really help you recognise when you are eating for emotional reasons rather than hunger. It can also help you be more aware of your full signal.

*Be realistic*

Even slim people give themselves treats occasionally. If you try to ban everything you enjoy, you're setting yourself up for failure. Don't be strict and unbending. A little of what you fancy isn't the end of the world. It's life!

*Recognise distortions*

If you can recognise when your brain is distorting your thoughts, you're in a position to tell it to stop. Brains hate change so it'll try to make you take the easy way out and do nothing. Take control and be the boss!

## Case Study: How I Took Back Control

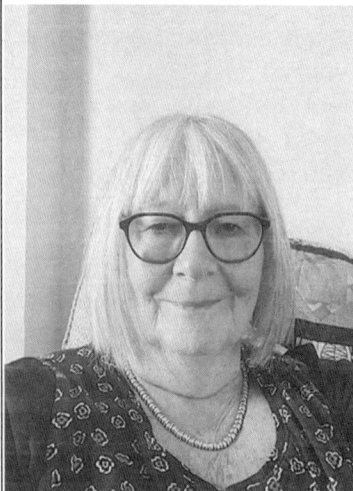

*Heather Manning*

For as long as I can remember, my weight has been a constant struggle. I've spent a lifetime being the 'bigger one' in my group of friends, never fully comfortable in my own skin. Over the years, I tried countless times to lose weight by dieting, with little success.

I wasn't obsessive, but it was always on my mind. I recall hitting my target weight once in those 40 years, and the joy was immense. But, like so many times before, it didn't last. Life's challenges, particularly the traumas, pushed me towards food for comfort.

Two years ago, when my son got married, I desperately wanted to lose weight for the wedding. I tried, I really did, but I didn't succeed. I remember feeling so disappointed in how I looked that day. As time went on, I grew more despondent.

I found myself buying size 24 clothes just to feel comfortable and that was a wake-up call. For my seventieth my daughter arranged for family photos at a beautiful castle. When I look at those pictures now, all I see is how unhappy I was with myself, even though everyone else saw me differently.

Then, one day, I came across Slimpod, and everything changed. From the very first day, I stopped snacking entirely. I no longer think about food until lunch or dinner. I've always eaten healthy meals, but my portions were too large. Now, I naturally eat smaller portions, and it's effortless. My body is changing, and so is my confidence. My knees and feet don't hurt as much anymore, and I'm looking forward to increasing my exercise this summer.

At 70, I feel like I'm coming back to life. I don't know how much weight I've lost because I threw away the scales. What I do know is that my clothes fit better, and I see a difference in the mirror.

These days, I feel in control. My confidence is returning in a way that feels genuine. I'm not constantly worrying about how I look anymore. Right now, I'm a size 18, and that feels absolutely wonderful to me. I know I'll be a size 16 soon enough, but I'm not stressed about when that will happen.

For the first time in a long time, I feel okay – truly okay – and that is something I didn't think was possible.

*Find out more about Heather's story here:*

## CHAPTER 17

# Tame Your Inner Critic, Transform Your Inner Voice

Over many years, one question has come up time and again within our Slimpod community: 'How do I stop negative self-talk from making me feel rubbish and sabotaging my efforts to lose weight?' Negative self-talk creates major mental health issues, and I'd love to help more people overcome it.

Most people know their inner critic really well. It's the voice in your head that judges you, doubts you, belittles you and constantly tells you you're not good enough. It says hurtful things to you – things you'd never say to another person, like: 'I am such an idiot', 'I am a fraud', 'I never do anything right' or 'I will never succeed.' People live with this for years and it does so much damage to their self-esteem. A lot of this comes from dieting over and over again, and blaming yourself for the diet not being successful, when actually it's not your fault.

Everything you say to yourself really matters. The inner critic is *not* harmless. It really does hold you back from enjoying the life you truly want to live. It robs you of peace of mind and emotional well-being, and, if left unchecked, it can even lead to serious mental health problems.

Self-criticism, instead of positive self-talk, is like choosing punishment over a reward. While punishment can sometimes work in the short term, rewards are generally better for shaping new and lasting behaviour.

When you punish yourself for what you do wrong, it doesn't teach you how to do it right. Imagine a small child learning to walk: if you screamed at them every time they fell down, you know that would have a negative impact. It would certainly have a very different effect than if you smiled and encouraged the child each time they took a step towards you.

When your inner critic consistently labels you in a negative way, it limits your self-belief and damages your self-esteem. Research suggests that negative thoughts tend to be stronger and more lasting than positive ones, making their impact profound and enduring.[1]

To take back control, you first need to be aware that these thoughts are going on. Much of our thinking is so automatic and happening so rapidly that we barely notice it before we move on to the next thought. Making the conscious effort to slow down and pay more attention to your inner dialogue will help you notice when the critic is present. Your emotions will also cue you to its presence. Negative emotions such as doubt, guilt, shame and worthlessness are almost always signs of the critic at work.

A good exercise to try for one week is to keep an inner critic log, either in a small notebook or on your phone. Every time you notice yourself being self-critical, just note down two or three words about the situation – for example, *got up late, meeting with boss, fight with Mum, lunch choices* – and what the criticism was – for example, *I'm lazy, I'm a bad employee, I'm not a good daughter, I have no self-control.* Once you are aware of the critical voice, you will be able to see if there's a pattern and begin the process of dealing with it.

The inner critic doesn't want you to notice it. It thrives best when you mistake it for being part of your identity. However, you weren't born with an inner critic. It's a voice you've internalised based on outside influences and learning, such as other people's criticism, expectations or standards. You adopt their limiting beliefs. This can be turned around, as research shows that recognising the critic as separate from yourself can reduce its negative impact.[2]

One way to do this is to give it the name of someone you really don't like very much or have no respect for. This means it immediately loses its power and you are on your way to freeing yourself from its influence.

Another strategy is to turn it from a harsh, critical voice into a more neutral or even supportive one. Imagine this voice is someone you respect or admire giving you advice. For example, instead of saying: 'You're such a failure', change it to: 'You made a mistake, but you can learn from this.' By altering the tone, you change the impact the voice has on you. This process can be incredibly empowering, transforming a source of negativity into a potential for growth.

Use your inner critic as a tool for improvement. Instead of letting it beat you down, engage with it like a coach. Early in my career, I questioned my self-worth and whether I was good enough. By changing the critic into a voice that gives constructive advice, I could start to see its potential for helping me grow.

Speak to yourself as if you were talking to a friend or mentor. For instance, say: 'Sandra, you know you're good at what you do, why are you doubting yourself?' This way, the inner critic becomes a guide rather than an obstacle.

Understanding the impact of the inner critic isn't just anecdotal. Numerous studies have explored how self-criticism affects mental health and behaviour. Research has shown that self-critical individuals are more likely to experience anxiety, depression and other mental health issues.[3]

By addressing and managing self-criticism, you can significantly improve your mental well-being and overall quality of life. Remember, the journey to taming your inner critic requires patience and persistence, but with time and effort, you can turn your inner voice into a powerful ally.

## How You Can Take Back Control

*Notice negative self-talk*

Be aware these thoughts are happening because that can help you understand and mitigate their impact. Keep a log of what the voice says so you can look for patterns.

*Give it a name*

Separate yourself from the critic by giving it a name, creating a visual image of someone you don't like or respect. See how doing this makes it lose its power. Do this every time it happens and it will soon disappear.

*Change the voice*

Instead of it being stern and critical, turn the voice into that of a supportive friend or coach. Make it someone you respect and admire; someone whose positive advice you value. Do this reframe every time your inner critic rears its head.

*Use it to grow*

Don't let the voice wear you down – use it as a tool for improvement. There's no failure, only feedback, so learn from the voice and use it as a guide not an obstacle.

## Case Study: How I Took Back Control

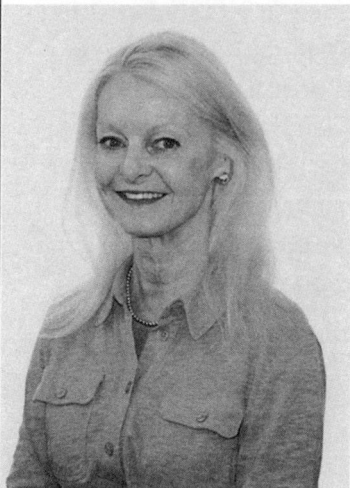

*Vivienne Chapman*

As the head teacher of a girls' school, I was constantly under the watchful eyes of 500 students every day. They noticed everything about me, from my make-up to my outfits. More than just their educator, I was a role model for how to navigate life, and that included learning about food and a healthy approach to body image.

In a world where social media can place unrealistic expectations on young women, I felt a profound responsibility to project a healthy relationship with food. But, deep down, I knew I wasn't living that example as well as I could.

I began teaching at 21 and, from then on, my life was a whirlwind of rushed meals, grabbed in between classes or while offering extra help to students. I rarely sat down to eat properly, always eating on the go, and never felt in control of my eating habits.

While I wasn't overweight, luckily, my relationship with food was anything but calm, and I knew I needed to change my approach, both for my sake and for the girls who looked up to me.

That's when I discovered Slimpod, and it truly transformed my mindset. I never thought I could go a day without chocolate, especially since I was denied sugar as a child and had developed a massive sweet tooth. But Slimpod helped me break that cycle. It was about trusting myself to make healthy choices naturally and ignore my inner critic, which said I'd never do it. This shift in mindset has been so valuable. Diets, I believe, can be toxic, especially for young people, setting them up for a lifetime of yo-yoing between weight loss and gain. I didn't want that for myself or the girls I was leading.

Now retired from the profession I loved, I find joy in the simplicity of healthy eating. I've always liked wholesome unprocessed foods, steamed and raw, but the constant lure of sugar was a challenge. Now, that craving has disappeared entirely. I no longer feel controlled by it, which has given me a new-found sense of calm. It's amazing how something as small as changing my approach to food has had such a ripple effect on my life.

The lessons I've learned not only improved my own life, but made me realise how important it is for teachers to have the tools to be better role models for the girls who are watching them every day.

This journey has been about more than just food – it's been about regaining control over my life and setting a positive example for others. Now, I feel so much calmer and better equipped to show everyone that they, too, can take control of their own lives, in a healthy, balanced way.

*Find out more about Vivienne's story here:*

## CHAPTER 18

# Rewire Your Habits: The Secret to Lasting Change

Consider this: you always tie the same shoelace first, automatically buckle your seatbelt when you get in the car and flinch when you hear a loud noise. These actions are seamless, almost robotic. How do they happen? That's the power of habits at work.

Habits streamline our repetitive tasks, conserving our brain's energy for more complex decisions. But how exactly do habits form, and why are they so powerful?

At the core of habit formation is the habit loop, consisting of three components:

1. **The trigger:** In neuroscience, what sets off a habit is called a stimulus, but I prefer to call it a trigger because it fires the gun that makes a habit kick in with the speed of a bullet. Triggers initiate the behaviour, and include things such as the time of day or an emotional state.
2. **The routine:** This is the behaviour itself.
3. **The reward:** This is the positive outcome you experience, reinforcing the habit loop.

When you do something that leads to a reward, your brain releases dopamine, creating a sense of pleasure. This 'feel-good' chemical reinforces the habit loop, making it more likely that you'll repeat the behaviour. Studies have shown that dopamine release is not just linked to the reward itself, but also to the anticipation of the reward. This anticipation helps establish and strengthen habits over time.[1]

Habits often run our lives without us even noticing. They're the reason you automatically grab a biscuit with your morning coffee or pour a glass of wine at the end of a long day. Many routines date back to childhood, where repetition ingrained them into our brains. Remember the endless reminders to 'look right, look left, look right again' before crossing the road or to wash your hands after using the toilet? These weren't just rules; they were training sessions for your brain, ensuring these actions became second nature.

Changing deeply ingrained habits can often feel like an uphill battle – believe me, I know. Most people on my Slimpod programme have spent more than 30 years trying and failing. However, with the right approach and mindset, turning challenging habits into rewarding ones that lead to a healthier, happier you is entirely achievable.

First, it's important to differentiate between reflex actions and habits. Reflexes are automatic responses hardwired from birth, like blinking when something approaches your eyes or jerking your hand away from a hot surface. These actions bypass the brain's conscious control, instead relying on a direct pathway through your nervous system.

Habits, on the other hand, are learned behaviours stored in a specific part of the brain. They require repetition to form but can be changed with a little effort. Research has discovered that the brain actually prefers new habits to old ones and, when habits are broken, they are not stored away but replaced with new ones.[2] The brain's preference for new habits is dynamite information for those struggling with eating and drinking habits. It means no one is stuck with bad habits forever.

Habits are triggered effortlessly and rapidly without awareness or intention so it's crucial to understand what sets yours off – like the time, a smell, a sound or a person.[3] For instance, you might not feel hungry at 8.30am but still find yourself eating a full English breakfast. You know cakes and biscuits make you gain weight, but elevenses and afternoon tea are part of everyday life. It's wine o'clock, pour me a large one. Make that two! You get the idea. These habits run in the background of your brain for years. Your habit finds a fleeting moment when your guard is down and kicks in because your ability to resist has suddenly switched off.[4]

This remarkable power of habits to disrupt your best intentions has been demonstrated across various health-related behaviours, including physical activity, sitting down for too long, what and how much you eat and drink, and even taking regular medication.[5] It's probably the main reason why dieting, or food deprivation as I call it, almost always fails however hard you try.

If you can interrupt these behaviour patterns by being aware of the triggers and how the habit process works, you're in with a great chance of changing things.

Once you can identify the cue that triggers a behaviour, you can then find a healthier routine that provides a similar reward. For example, if stress (trigger) leads you to snack on junk food (routine), you might replace this with a brief walk or deep breathing exercise (new routine) that still offers stress relief (reward).[6]

## Bend Your Mind to Break Hard Habits

With persistence and the right techniques, you can also harness the power of neuroplasticity (see page 108) and teach your brain to find pleasure in habits that initially seem difficult. Consistency is the key here. Research shows that the repeated practice of a new skill leads to structural changes in the brain, embedding new behaviours more deeply into your daily routine.[7]

James Clear, author of *Atomic Habits*, emphasises the importance of small changes in building new habits. He introduced the concept of 'one per cent better every day', suggesting that tiny improvements can lead to significant long-term results. B.J. Fogg, a behaviour scientist at Stanford University and author of *Tiny Habits*, offers a similar perspective. He says successful habit formation starts with tiny actions that are easy to perform. For example, if you want to develop a habit of flossing, start by flossing just one tooth. This tiny action is manageable, reducing the barrier to entry and increasing the likelihood of consistency.[8]

So, the first step is breaking down hard habits into smaller, more manageable steps. This approach, often referred to as 'micro-habits', allows you to build confidence and momentum gradually. For instance, if you want to develop a habit of exercising regularly but find it challenging, start with just five minutes a day. As this becomes a routine, gradually increase the duration and intensity. Research also highlights the effectiveness of starting small to reduce resistance and build positive momentum.[9]

Positive reinforcement is another powerful tool. Reward yourself in a helpful way immediately after completing a hard new habit. Positive reinforcement encourages your brain to associate the challenging activity with a sense of satisfaction and pleasure. A study on dopamine and reward mechanisms shows how positive reinforcement strengthens neural pathways associated with desired behaviours, making them more likely to stick.[10] These rewards don't have to be extravagant; they can be simple things like taking a relaxing bath or spending a few minutes on a hobby you love. Somebody I know gets a dopamine kick by putting a £1 coin in a pot every time she wants to reward herself for not eating chocolate – and it really adds up. She's bought all sorts of things with the money and it gives her an incredible buzz!

Visualisation is equally important. Spend a few minutes each day imagining yourself successfully completing the new habit and experiencing the positive outcomes it brings. For example, if you're trying to develop a habit of waking up early, visualise yourself waking up feeling refreshed, having a productive morning and enjoying the benefits of an early start. Visualisation helps create a mental blueprint for success, making the habit feel more attainable and enjoyable.[11] We'll explore this in more detail in Chapter 26.

Another crucial strategy is to regularly remind yourself of the long-term benefits associated with the new habit. Keeping your eye on the bigger picture can help you stay motivated during challenging moments. Write down the positive changes you expect to see and refer to this list whenever you feel discouraged. For example, if you're working on eating more healthily, focus on the increased energy, better mood and improved well-being you'll enjoy as a result. By keeping these benefits at the forefront of your mind, you can shift your focus from the immediate difficulty to the rewarding outcomes.

Retraining your brain to break old habits requires patience, persistence and self-compassion. It's important to celebrate small victories along the way and be kind to yourself when you encounter setbacks. Remember that progress, not perfection, is the goal. The old saying is wrong: practice doesn't make perfect – it makes better. And better is enough because better is success.

However hard it is at first, each small step forward is a triumph that brings you closer to making the new habit a natural and enjoyable part of your life. So embrace the power of your mind to adapt and grow. Believe in your ability to transform challenging habits into sources of joy and fulfilment. With time, effort and the right strategies, you can rewire your brain not only to accept, but also to enjoy the habits that lead to a healthier, happier you. I know you can do this!

Remember, the power to change lies within you, and every small step brings you closer to your goals.

## How You Can Take Back Control

*Identify the cue*

Recognise what triggers your habit. Is it a specific time of day, an emotional state or a particular environment?

*Alter the reward*

Replace the unwanted behaviour with a healthier one. Choose actions that are easy and rewarding.

*Celebrate new habits*

Ensure the new behaviour provides a satisfying outcome. This reinforcement will help solidify the new habit.

*Start small for big success*

Begin with manageable steps to build confidence and momentum. For example, if exercise is daunting, start with five minutes a day and gradually increase.

*Reward your efforts*

Reinforce new habits with positive rewards. Enjoy a favourite healthy snack or hobby to associate the habit with pleasure.

*Visualise future success*

Spend time each day visualising the positive outcomes of your new habit. Imagine the benefits and let this mental blueprint guide you (see Chapter 26 for more guidance on visualisation).

# Case Study: How I Took Back Control

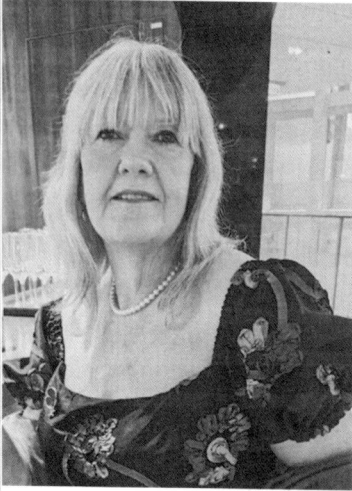

*Lyn Fox*
I'd lost weight and put it on again umpteen times, as we do in the yo-yo dieting world, and I had issues with my knees because I wasn't exercising. We moved into a new house just before Covid and it had stairs up to the bedrooms and down to another lounge. I told my husband, 'I don't think I can stay here. We'll have to move.' I was really worried one of my knees would go and I'd fall down the stairs.

Then a friend sent me a photograph of myself and it was horrendous. I was about 32kg (five stone) overweight. I knew I had to do something. And as if by magic an ad popped up on Facebook for Slimpod.

From the very start, I absolutely loved it. I found myself being in control again and wanting to eat healthier foods, like hummus and tomatoes. Weird! I'd hated the smell of tomatoes since childhood. But suddenly, I loved them and my whole diet became much healthier. My family's did, too.

A few weeks later I had a hospital appointment for my knees and the doctor gave me painkillers for osteoarthritis. But the packet is still unopened because, as I lost weight, the pain in my knees went away. So far I've lost all of that 32kg and more.

The lighter me does a seven-minute workout in the mornings using a video on YouTube, and I can climb the stairs again. In fact, I've embraced exercise so much that I have a personal trainer and I've started to do strength exercises like squats with weights. I'm running my life now, not my knees! I do a lot of walking and I've gone back to Zumba classes again. Before, I was doing exercise for the wrong reasons – to try to lose weight. Now I do it because I want to and I enjoy it; it's part of who I am now. Amazing.

We're going on a cruise soon and 18 months ago I would have booked it solely because they had a 24-hour buffet. Now I've already booked my gym tickets on board. That's not the person I used to be.

My life's just totally, totally different. I saw somebody the other day struggling to walk down the road and I thought, 'Wow, I was like that only 18 months ago.' Now I don't just walk up the stairs – I run up them. See, it can be done!

*Find out more about Lyn's story here:*

# CHAPTER 19

# Unlock the Power of Anchors

In my years of helping people achieve sustainable weight loss, one concept has stood out as both incredibly powerful and often overlooked: the science and psychology of anchors. Anchors are stimuli that create unconscious habits, shaping our behaviours in ways we often don't realise.

Understanding and harnessing this power can be a game changer. Anchors are like invisible strings that tie certain stimuli to automatic responses. They can be anything from a specific smell to a particular time of day, and they trigger behaviours without us even being aware of it.

This concept is rooted in classical conditioning, a type of learning discovered by Ivan Pavlov in the early twentieth century. Pavlov found that dogs could be trained to salivate at the sound of a bell if the sound was repeatedly paired with the presentation of food.[1] This basic principle extends far beyond dogs and bells. Human brains are constantly forming associations between different stimuli and responses. For example, if you always snack while watching TV, your brain starts to link the two activities. Eventually, just sitting down in front of the TV can make you crave a snack, even if you're not hungry. This is an anchor at work.

The power of anchors lies in their ability to create unconscious habits. These are behaviours that are performed automatically because they have been repeated in a consistent context.[2] This means that if you can identify and change the anchors in your life, you can significantly alter your habits and, consequently, your weight.

Imagine you have a habit of eating biscuits every afternoon. This habit likely started with an anchor – perhaps the time of day or a particular feeling of boredom or stress. Each time you ate a biscuit in response to this anchor, the connection in your brain grew stronger. Over time, the anchor and the behaviour became so tightly linked that you now find yourself reaching for biscuits without even thinking about it. Breaking this cycle involves identifying the anchor and replacing the associated behaviour with a healthier one.

For instance, if 3 p.m. is your usual biscuit time, you could plan to have a cup of herbal tea instead. By consistently pairing 3 p.m. with tea rather than biscuits, you'll gradually weaken the old anchor and strengthen a new, healthier one.

This process is supported by the brain's ability to reorganise itself by forming new neural connections – the concept of neuroplasticity that we've already explored.[3] This means that no matter how ingrained your current habits are, you have the power to change them.

Anchors don't just apply to eating habits, of course. They can influence all sorts of behaviours that impact your weight. For example, if you tend to skip workouts because you associate exercise with discomfort or failure, you can create new anchors that make exercise a positive experience. Start by setting a consistent time for your workouts and pair them with something you enjoy, like listening to your favourite music or exercising with a friend. Over time, these positive associations will make it easier to stick with your fitness routine.

Another fascinating aspect of anchors is their ability to affect our emotional responses. This is particularly relevant for emotional eaters who turn to food for comfort. A study found that people often eat in response to negative emotions because food provides a temporary distraction and sense of pleasure.[4] By recognising the emotional anchors that trigger your eating, you can start to address the underlying issues and find healthier ways to cope. For instance, if stress at work leads you to binge on junk food, identify that stress as your anchor. Then, develop alternative responses that don't involve eating. This might include taking a short walk, practising deep breathing exercises or even just stepping away from your desk for a few minutes. The key is to create a new, positive behaviour that you can consistently turn to when you feel stressed.

It's also worth noting that not all anchors are negative. You can intentionally create positive anchors to support your weight-loss goals – for example, placing your running shoes by the door as a visual reminder to exercise or keeping a water bottle on your desk to encourage hydration. These small changes can make a big difference by constantly nudging you towards healthier choices.

In my experience, the most successful weight-loss journeys are those that embrace the power of anchors. By reshaping the associations in your brain, you can transform your habits and create a healthier, happier life. It's about working with your brain's natural tendencies rather than against them, and, with patience and persistence, you can achieve your goals.

By understanding and leveraging the power of anchors, you can make meaningful and lasting changes to your habits. This knowledge equips you to navigate your weight-loss journey with greater awareness and control, ultimately leading to a healthier and more fulfilling life.

Remember, this is not about perfection, but about making gradual, consistent changes that lead to lasting results.

---

## How You Can Take Back Control

### Swap negative anchors

Start by pinpointing the triggers for your unhealthy habits. If you always reach for a snack at a set time, swap sweet stuff for a healthier option. By consistently pairing the same time with a better choice, you'll reprogramme your brain to crave the healthier option.

### Pair exercise with enjoyment

Make workouts a positive experience by linking them with something you love. Set a consistent workout time. Do something you enjoy at the end, like sitting in a park or having a skinny latte, because this creates positive associations.

### Create visual reminders

Use visual cues to constantly nudge you towards healthy behaviours. Place your running shorts and top by the bed at night so you see them when you wake up. Save a selfie of yourself out jogging as your phone's wallpaper.

---

## CHAPTER 20

# Overcome Guilt – The Silent Saboteur

Three-quarters of women in the UK – a staggering 24 million – frequently experience guilt over how much they eat. On average, women think about food 12 times a day – that's 46,000 times in their lifetime.[1] This statistic reveals a profound issue that touches the lives of millions, yet it often goes unaddressed in conversations about healthy living.

The problem isn't just about feeling bad after eating a piece of chocolate or a bag of crisps; it's a deeper, more pervasive issue that can significantly affect your approach to weight loss and well-being.

Guilt is a natural, ingrained response to doing something you consider to be wrong. It's drummed into us by parents, teachers and societal norms. Food guilt is triggered when you label foods as inherently 'good' or 'bad', often a residue from years of stressful, failed dieting. Unfortunately, putting a moral value on what you eat means you're inevitably also passing moral judgement on yourself for eating it.

It's crucial to understand the impact of this kind of thinking on your soul. Over time, it can lead you into a damaging cycle of self-blame: 'Eating bad chocolate means I'm a bad person. I hate myself.' It makes me so sad whenever someone confesses this to me. Here's what I tell them: everyone indulges in treats every now and then – it's called living! And actually, if you want to lose weight, being too strict about every morsel that passes your lips can sabotage your goals, not to mention your self-esteem. As I've said before, when it comes down to it, weight loss is about much more than the food you eat. It's important to consider your overall well-being.

The most important advice I can give you is to pay attention to your body, treat yourself well and, above all, be kind to yourself. Dealing with food guilt is a crucial part of this.

The worst thing about food guilt is how quickly it spirals out of control. If you're 'being good' on a diet and then suddenly eat something you've labelled as naughty or bad, you might think you've blown it all and tend to eat even more. Some experts call this the 'what-the-hell' effect. Dieters call it falling off the wagon. This cycle of catastrophising can lead to you consuming far more food and calories than if you just allowed yourself a treat without the guilt.

By giving the treat a meaning that becomes emotionally charged, feelings can take over from rational thought and the result is self-sabotage and hindering your weight-loss progress. But no food is inherently good or bad – there are just foods that are healthier than others.

Psychological studies suggest that when we associate eating with guilt, we're more likely to experience stress, which can lead to overeating.[2] This is detrimental not only to our weight-loss goals, but also to our self-esteem and mental health. The relentless pursuit of dietary perfection often leads to a black-and-white view of eating, where foods are either completely off-limits or consumed excessively once 'allowed'. This can create an unhealthy relationship with food, where eating becomes a source of anxiety rather than nourishment.[3]

Understanding the roots of food anxiety involves delving into the brain's mechanisms and the psychological impact of dieting. Restrictive diets often result in heightened food cravings and increased anxiety about eating.[4] This anxiety stems from the fear of breaking the diet and the potential consequences; when your brain senses this potential for failure, it goes into a heightened state of alert, making every food choice feel like a critical decision. Labelling foods as off-limits can make them more desirable, leading to a cycle of restriction, anxiety and binge eating.[5] When we label foods as 'bad', we not only crave them more, but also feel intense guilt when we inevitably give in to these cravings.

Our brains learn through experiences, much like a scientist collecting data. Each positive or negative experience with food adds to our beliefs and attitudes towards eating. If you continuously restrict and fear certain foods, your brain strengthens the association between food and anxiety. Avoidance only serves to reinforce fear. By not confronting the foods you fear, you never give your brain the opportunity to learn that these foods are not inherently harmful. This avoidance can trap you in a cycle of anxiety and fear.

Research shows that exposure to feared stimuli in a controlled manner can reduce anxiety over time.[6] This principle applies to food fears as well: confronting and consuming feared foods can help diminish anxiety. By repeatedly exposing yourself to these foods in a controlled way, you can teach your brain that there is no real danger.

Consider these four ways to take back control:

### Practise exposure therapy

Gradually introduce feared foods into your diet in small, manageable amounts. This exposure helps your brain learn that these foods are not harmful, reducing anxiety over time. Start with less intimidating foods and gradually work your way up to those that cause more fear. This helps to systematically desensitise your brain to the fear-inducing foods.

### Challenge negative thoughts

When you think, 'I can't eat this, it's bad', reframe it to: 'This food can nourish my body and fit into a balanced lifestyle.' Acknowledging that all foods can have a place in moderation helps reduce the black-and-white thinking that fuels anxiety. By questioning these negative thoughts, you weaken their hold on your behaviour.

### Adopt a flexible eating approach

Flexible, or intuitive, eating helps you to listen to your body's natural hunger and fullness cues, fostering a more balanced approach to food. It's important that you don't count calories or ban certain foods. Eat smaller amounts of what you know is healthy, but have the occasional small treat if you fancy it. This reduces the pressure and anxiety associated with strict dietary rules. Research on intuitive eating supports the benefits of this approach.[7]

**Seek support from others**

Surround yourself with a supportive community. Sharing your experiences and receiving guidance can provide the encouragement and strategies needed to overcome food anxiety. This helps you to feel less isolated and more empowered to make positive changes.

Breaking free from the clutches of food guilt involves a significant shift in mindset. It's about recognising that occasional indulgence is part of a balanced life and not a moral failing. I know you can do it!

## How You Can Take Back Control

### Start viewing food as neutral

Foods aren't 'good' or 'bad'; they simply have different nutritional values. This mindset can prevent feelings of guilt and help you to maintain a more balanced diet. Instead of dividing food into good and bad camps, develop the attitude that you can have all food in moderation.

### Engage with the eating experience

Pay more attention to the flavours, textures and sensations of your food. Mindfulness helps in recognising when you are physically hungry versus emotionally driven to eat, reducing instances where guilt might take over.[8]

### Don't try to be perfect

A treat is part of normal eating; nothing bad is going to happen. Unlike an all-or-nothing attitude, thinking this way helps you rein in the 'falling off the wagon' effect. Remember, moderation is key, and enjoying an occasional treat can be part of a healthy diet.[9]

### Talk kindly to yourself

Research has shown that adopting a more compassionate approach to eating can lead to better weight management outcomes and improved psychological well-being.[10] By shifting our focus from guilt to acceptance, we can enjoy a more balanced, fulfilling approach to eating. Replace negative self-talk with kinder, more forgiving messages. Remind yourself that it's okay to enjoy food and that one treat doesn't ruin your progress. Self-compassion can reduce stress and prevent the cycle of guilt and overeating.

## Case Study: How I Took Back Control

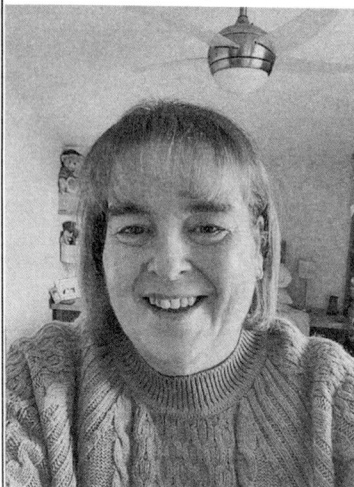

*Clare Rayner*

Two years ago, I made a list of three things I no longer wanted in my life: to end up in a wheelchair, to suffer from constant boils and to be woken by the pain of pins and needles every night because my weight was cutting off circulation to my arms. At the time, I was a size 26/28, eating mindlessly and dealing with random heart palpitations.

Even something as simple as cutting my toenails felt like an adventure. I was bitter, sad and in constant pain from my aching knees. Walking my beloved dog was becoming nearly impossible. I was pretending to count calories, but felt utterly hopeless. I was also avoiding my husband's work friends because I was too ashamed of my appearance.

Fast-forward to now, and everything has changed. I've gone from a size 28 to an 18, but what I've gained is far more significant than the dress sizes I've lost. I now have the confidence to wear a short dress and enjoy my day without a second thought.

The freedom I've found through this journey is immeasurable and should never be underestimated. I no longer worry about what my daughters might say about my clothing choices. What truly matters is how I feel about myself.

The three things on my list are now distant memories. I can't recall the last time I was woken by pins and needles. Today, I'm a size 18 and, just last weekend, I bought a size 16 dress. It's a flowy number, but it fits, and there was no way I wasn't buying it!

Without thinking about it, I've become an intermittent faster. I swim sixty-four lengths three times a week, work out twice a week, run twice a week and walk my dog three times a day. I've cut out crisps and chocolate and now eat mainly the Mediterranean way because it's delicious. Most importantly, I'm happy, confident and have finally met one of my husband's friends, with plans to meet more soon.

I still have weight to lose, and I'm confident I will over the next year. By making good food choices, moving more and focusing on the blessings in my life instead of envying others, I'm in a better place.

For me, the biggest win is my mindset. The positivity I have now is incredible. I used to worry about what people thought, but now I wear dresses and don't care what others think. My mindset has transformed completely, allowing me to enjoy life without guilt or fear.

*Find out more about Clare's story here:*

## CHAPTER 21

# Stop Your Mind Fighting Against You

Now we're going to delve into the little-known yet crucial concept that we touched on earlier: cognitive dissonance – the silent saboteur that plays a significant role in your weight-loss journey. This psychological phenomenon occurs when there's a clash between what you consciously decide to do and what your subconscious, deep-down beliefs and values want to do.

For example, you may consciously decide to eat healthier food, exercise more or reduce your sugar intake. But subconsciously, there could be deeply rooted beliefs that contradict these decisions. You may have learned to associate relaxation with a glass of wine or believe that sweets are a reward for a tough day. This belief system, nestled in your subconscious, then wages a silent battle against your conscious efforts to change.

Cognitive dissonance in the realm of eating habits and weight loss is particularly stealthy – it creeps up silently, with a guise of comfort, but deep down it's in disarray, a conflict that can disrupt your best-laid plans for a healthier lifestyle.

Bear in mind that the subconscious mind is the power behind everything you do. From breathing to blinking, it ensures that many tasks are performed efficiently, allowing your conscious mind to focus on more complex activities. When it comes to eating, your subconscious is shaped by years of learned behaviours, emotional associations and habitual responses. As we saw in Chapter 18, habits are formed through neuroplasticity, where repeated behaviours create and strengthen neural pathways in the brain.

Once a habit is established, it becomes automatic, freeing up mental resources for other tasks. This is why you might find yourself reaching for a snack without even thinking about it. Your brain has linked certain cues – like feeling stressed or watching TV – with the routine of eating, followed by the reward of satisfaction or comfort.

When you start a diet, you're essentially trying to override these automatic behaviours with conscious effort. Diets often require you to monitor what you eat, count calories and follow strict rules. This conscious control is in direct conflict with the effortless, automatic nature of your subconscious habits. It's no wonder this feels like a constant battle!

Cognitive dissonance is not just an academic term; it's a daily reality for many, and is often a hurdle that can hinder weight loss.

Picture the internal tug-of-war that happens when you resolve not to eat sweets, only to weaken and rationalise later that 'just one won't hurt'. Or when you promise yourself to exercise to offset an indulgent meal, yet find excuses not to.[1] These mental gymnastics are all symptoms of cognitive dissonance – your brain's struggle to hold two opposing thoughts at the same time. The subconscious mind is incredibly powerful and, often, our desires stem from it, overshadowing our conscious decisions. The solution is not to mute the conversation between your conscious and subconscious, but to foster a dialogue between them, to align your beliefs with your actions.

This is what sets mind-retraining programmes like Slimpod apart: they work to harmonise your conscious goals with your subconscious drivers, making the journey towards healthier habits feel less like climbing a mountain and more like a gentle walk in the park.

The key to bridging the gap between the subconscious and conscious mind is awareness. Many people struggle because they're unaware of the subconscious beliefs that hold them back. By shining a light on these hidden beliefs, you can begin to unravel them.

Deconstructing and disputing the belief is key, so start by asking yourself some reflective questions:

- What do I believe?
- Are these beliefs true and based on facts?
- How do these beliefs affect my feelings and behaviours?
- Are they serving my current weight-loss goals and well-being?

If you suspect sugar is your nemesis, ask what emotional need it fulfils. Is it comfort, reward, a source of energy or something else? For alcohol, is it about relaxation? That's the case for so many people. Then question whether it truly relaxes you, or is it just a long-held belief?

Dig down a bit deeper. Think about where this belief may have come from and, more importantly, why it's become a belief that you feel is true. It's crucial to uncover the actual truths about your beliefs and see them for what they are. By challenging these beliefs, you start to weaken their hold on you.

You can do this by turning the belief on its head. For example: 'I might get a real high from the initial effects of sugar or alcohol, but then I feel bad, feel guilty and even feel a failure – it does nothing for me apart from cause anxiety and stress.'

Then go further with this rationalisation. Think of all the counterproductive and unhelpful things that happen as a result of what you've consumed.

After you've done this you can then be objective about whether the original belief is still serving a purpose for you or not. It's a great exercise in getting out of your own way!

But overcoming cognitive dissonance is not an overnight fix. It's about finding clarity in your intentions, understanding the underlying reasons for your actions and reshaping your thoughts to foster a congruent, harmonious mind.[2]

Recognising and dealing with this dissonance can pivot your journey from one of struggle to one of harmony. Ingrained habits and beliefs are not immutable laws of nature; they're malleable. Understanding that your subconscious habits are powerful doesn't mean you're doomed to fail. Instead, it offers insight into how you can approach weight loss more effectively.

## How You Can Take Back Control

*Tune into your thoughts*

Start by becoming an observer of your own mind. When you feel the urge to eat something you know doesn't align with your goals, pause and reflect on what's driving this desire. Is it hunger, habit, emotion or a deep-seated belief?

*Challenge your truths*

Question the 'truths' you hold about food. Are they based on evidence or are they simply beliefs passed down or formed from past experiences? Write them down and scrutinise them critically to create your very own belief busters.

*Align your actions and values*

Strive for congruence between what you value and what you do. If health is a core value, align your actions accordingly. Make choices that resonate with this value, and you'll find the dissonance being replaced by a sense of integrity and purpose.

*Embrace change gradually*

Overwhelming yourself with drastic changes can heighten cognitive dissonance. Instead, take small, manageable baby steps towards your goal. Gradual change can help reconcile your subconscious with your new reality, making the transition smoother and more sustainable.

*Reinforce new beliefs*

Every time you make a choice that supports your weight-loss goals, you're reinforcing a new belief system. Celebrate these moments. Write down your wins. Consistent confirmation of your new habits gradually remodels your subconscious beliefs.

## Case Study: How I Took Back Control

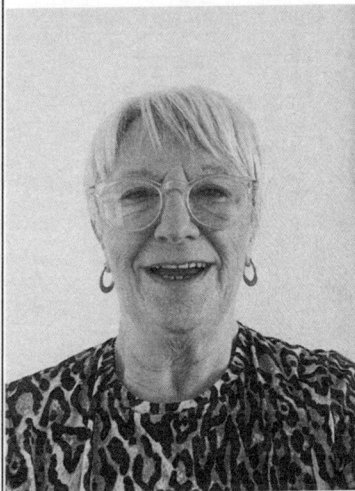

*Ronnie Gregory*

I was a constant snacker with a serious love for chips, muffins and chocolate. I'd tried countless diets, but nothing ever seemed to last for long. I felt stuck, trapped by my own cravings, and overwhelmed by the thought of changing.

But here I am, four years later and 20kg (3st) lighter. My journey wasn't instant, and it didn't start smoothly. It took a long time for my brain to get into gear, but, once it did, everything changed.

I realised that my struggles weren't just about food; they were about mindset. I'd been carrying around years of diet head mentality that was holding me back, but I finally found a way to let go of that.

What really made a difference was when I stopped thinking of food as 'good' or 'bad'. I stopped dieting and started listening to my body. I began to understand what it truly needed, and that's when the weight started coming off. Instead of feeling like I had to swap chips for salads, I wanted to. It wasn't about restriction anymore; it was about making choices that made me feel good.

For me, the real breakthrough came when I relaxed and let go of the pressure. I used to stress over every muffin, feeling guilty if I indulged. But once I realised that it was okay to enjoy a treat every now and then, something clicked. I didn't feel deprived anymore, and the pounds started to melt away. It was as if giving myself permission to enjoy food actually helped me control it better.

Taking control of my life wasn't just about losing weight. It was about reclaiming my confidence and happiness. Now, when I go out for a meal, I don't feel like I have to order a burger and chips just because it's there. Sometimes, I genuinely want a salad, and that's what I order. It's not about willpower; it's about what I truly want.

Even my relationship with exercise has changed. I started going to the gym with my daughter, something that was unheard of for me before. Now I go twice a week, and I actually enjoy it. It's become part of my routine, something I look forward to.

This journey has been about learning to trust myself again, about finding balance and joy in the choices I make. I'm finally in control, and it feels amazing.

*Find out more about Ronnie's story here:*

# CHAPTER 22

# Avoid the Willpower Trap

This statistic may surprise you: the average person thinks about food 200 times every day[1] and spends four hours a day using willpower to resist temptation.[2]

When starting a new weight-loss regime, most people rely heavily on willpower, but this is the very thing that often lets them down and sabotages all their hard work. I prefer to call willpower 'won't power' – 'I won't eat this and I won't eat that' – but it never works for long, does it?

Every day I hear people say, 'I have no willpower and that's why I can't lose weight,' blaming themselves for not being able to stick to their weight-loss efforts. When they do this repeatedly, they feel like failures. But now you're going to learn something that will change all this, and you'll no longer feel frustrated, miserable or a failure.

You see, willpower is commonly believed to be the constant driver of change. But if you peel back the layers, you'll find that willpower is more like a reservoir than an endless stream – it's finite and it can run dry.[3] Willpower – or self-control to give it another name – is the ability to resist short-term temptations to achieve long-term goals. It requires conscious thought and effort. However, as we discovered in the previous chapter when we looked at cognitive dissonance, the conscious mind is in a constant battle with the unconscious mind – the feelings and thoughts you have without being aware of them and which influence the way you behave.

Here's an example: you vow that you're never going to eat a sugar-laden custard tart again. That's a conscious decision. After a day or two (sometimes only an hour or two!), your unconscious mind starts planting unhelpful thoughts in your head: *I really love custard tarts; Custard tarts make me feel happy; Not eating them is making me sad; I'm sure just one wouldn't hurt me, and once I feel happy again, it will be easier to stop eating them.* Despite all your best intentions, will-power eventually loses and custard tarts win.

Relying solely on willpower to change eating habits or curb alcohol intake is building a house on shaky ground. Neuroscientists understand that willpower operates on a limited reserve of mental energy. As this is used up, it reduces our capacity to maintain self-control and willpower tends to pack up and leave.[4]

One fascinating study illustrated this by showing how participants who resisted chocolate biscuits for 15 minutes and ate healthy radishes instead then displayed less perseverance on subsequent tasks, suggesting their self-control resources had been drained.[5]

So the more you consciously fight the urge to overeat all the wrong things, the more your willpower runs out – until, eventually, you can't resist any longer and have to give in to that persuasive inner voice of temptation. Like everything in life, the brain is at the centre of it all.

Let's dig a little deeper into what happens when you're using your conscious mind and willpower to try to control what you eat. People who rely on their subconscious hunger signal to manage their eating are called intuitive eaters and those, like dieters, who try to use willpower are called controlled eaters. The interesting thing is that intuitive eaters are less likely to be overweight, and they spend less time thinking about food.

Controlled eaters are more vulnerable to overeating in response to advertising or temptations in supermarkets and coffee shops. And a small indulgence, like eating one scoop of ice cream, is more likely to lead to a food binge in controlled eaters.

Children are especially vulnerable to this cycle of dieting and then bingeing. Several long-term studies have shown that girls who diet in their early teenage years are three times more likely to become overweight five years later.[6]

Why is this? First of all, depriving yourself of something you like means your brain automatically desires it more. I'm sure you've noticed this! If you can't have cake, then that's all you see and want! Research has demonstrated that our actions are more driven by immediate emotions and desires than distant rewards.[7] Plus, the stress of having to make constant conscious decisions when you're on a diet disrupts the brain's impulse-control mechanisms, making the instant gratification of a cake more enticing than the long-term benefits of a slimmer waistline.[8]

Secondly, our environment is really not set up to help us lose weight. There are unhealthy food temptations everywhere. Every supermarket is stacked with processed ready meals full of hidden sugar; every high street is lined with junk food takeaway outlets.

Everyday life is one decision after another: what to wear, what to eat for breakfast, which route to work to take, which emails to open, which ones to answer, which phone calls to take, what time to have lunch, when to look at social media, what to buy for dinner, whether to help the kids with their homework, what story to read them at bedtime . . . The list is endless and exhausting.

Every decision drains your willpower battery and uses up precious resources of glucose, the fuel your brain runs on. No wonder that at the end of the day you're suffering from decision fatigue.[9] How often do you slump in a chair and say: 'That's it! I can't decide another thing'? Your ability to make a healthy choice for dinner or to have just one glass of wine instead of three is now non-existent. Willpower has wilted. Weight loss is out of the window. Your brain has abandoned you and old habits kick in.

So how do you get around the willpower problem? What's the alternative?

Retraining your brain to bypass the need for conscious self-control is the key and that means enlisting the support of the subconscious – your automatic brain.

Most of what you do every day is automatic, like cleaning your teeth, driving your car and even putting one foot in front of the other to walk. You had to learn how to do all those things, but when you'd done them a number of times, you no longer had to think about them and they became part of your day-to-day automatic behaviour.

Once that part of your brain is on your side, there is no need for willpower. Consistent healthy eating becomes your default mode, an automatic habit that requires no thinking, no decisions, no effort. And that's the key factor in achieving a new lifestyle that makes weight loss stress-free and sustainable.

## How You Can Take Back Control

### Plan and prepare meals

Create a shopping list, then plan and prepare your healthy meals in advance. I know a lot of people who batch-cook/prep on a Sunday for the whole week. Having healthy options readily available reduces the need to make decisions when you're tired and more likely to give in to temptation.

### Change the environment

Remove unhealthy snacks from your home and workplace. Surround yourself with healthy food choices to make it easier to stick to your goals.

### Establish a routine

Consistency is key. Set regular times for meals and exercise to build habits that become really easy and automatic. This reduces the need for willpower as your body adjusts to a predictable schedule.

### Focus on small changes

Instead of drastic dieting, make small, sustainable changes to your eating habits. Gradual adjustments are more likely to become permanent behaviours, reducing the reliance on willpower.

# CHAPTER 23

# Sidestep the Influence of Marketing Tricks

Hands up if you're a sucker for a BOGOF (buy one get one free) offer, meal deals or things which are placed right beside the cash desks in the supermarkets! Have you noticed that the sweets/crisps/alcohol are towards the end of your natural journey through the supermarket?

They are deliberately placed there because the supermarket knows that, by the end of a shopping visit (especially if you have children with you), you are at your most vulnerable and need a boost. Wham – you go for the treats!

Marketers are masters of unconscious persuasion, skilfully using subtle cues and psychological tactics to influence your decisions without you even realising it. They tap into your subconscious mind, shaping your perceptions and behaviours in ways that feel almost effortless.[1] This behind-the-scenes influence can have a profound impact on your choices, especially when it comes to purchasing food products.

Imagine walking into a supermarket and immediately feeling drawn to a particular brand of cereal. You might think it's because you like the taste or have heard good things about it. However, what you don't realise is that the marketer has strategically designed every aspect of that cereal box to appeal to your subconscious mind. From the colours used to the placement on the shelf, every detail is carefully crafted to grab your attention and persuade you to make a purchase.[2]

One of the most effective tools in a marketer's arsenal is the fascinating psychological principle of priming.

## How priming influences weight loss

Priming subtly yet powerfully influences your thoughts, behaviours and decisions. Understanding priming can offer profound insights into how you can harness it to support your weight-loss journey and overall well-being.

Priming is the process by which exposure to a stimulus influences your response to a subsequent stimulus, without conscious guidance or intention. In simpler terms, priming is like planting a seed in your mind that affects how you perceive and react to things later on.[3] This seed can be anything from a word or image, to a smell or even a concept. Once planted, it subtly shapes your thoughts and actions, often without you realising it.

For instance, if you read the word 'happy', you're more likely to notice and engage with positive, joyful things in your environment shortly afterwards. Similarly, if you see images of healthy foods and fit individuals, you might feel more motivated to make healthier choices yourself.

One study demonstrated how priming could affect behaviour.[4] Participants primed with words related to old age walked more slowly than those who were not. This shows how subtle cues can significantly influence your actions and decisions.

Priming can be used to nudge consumers towards a particular product. For instance, if you've seen adverts for a specific brand of cereal throughout the week, you're more likely to notice and choose that brand when you're at the store. The constant exposure primes your brain to associate positive feelings with that brand, making it a more appealing choice when you're faced with a decision.[5]

Priming plays a significant role in your eating habits and can either help or hinder your efforts to maintain a healthy lifestyle.

Conflict can arise when your conscious intentions to eat healthily clash with the subconscious cues you've absorbed from marketing tactics. You might consciously decide to avoid sugary snacks, but after seeing numerous advertisements, you might find yourself craving and eventually buying that chocolate bar. You might consciously decide to eat a salad for lunch, but the smell of a nearby pizza shop triggers a craving for something less healthy. This internal conflict can make it challenging to stick to your health goals.

By intentionally surrounding yourself with positive, health-promoting cues, you can use priming to your advantage.

Be mindful of the media you consume and choose sources that inspire and motivate you. Watching shows or reading articles that emphasise healthy living can prime you to adopt similar behaviours. On the other hand, constant exposure to content that glorifies indulgence and unhealthy eating can undermine your efforts.[6]

The people we interact with also act as primes. Conversations with friends who prioritise their health can motivate you to do the same, while spending time with those who have unhealthy habits can lead you astray.[7] Seek out relationships and communities that support and reinforce your healthy lifestyle choices.

Remember, the changes you seek often start with small, seemingly insignificant shifts in your mindset and environment. By harnessing the power of priming, you can create a supportive framework that makes healthy choices feel natural and effortless.

### The persuasive power of colours

Another powerful example of unconscious persuasion is the use of colours. Marketers know that certain colours evoke specific emotions and reactions. For instance, red can create a sense of urgency and excitement, which is why it's often used in clearance sales and promotional signs.[8] On the other hand, green is associated with health and tranquillity, making it a popular choice for brands that want to convey natural and organic qualities. By using these colour associations, marketers can subtly guide your feelings and decisions without you even being aware of it.

Research shows how colours can impact mood and behaviour. It found that red enhances performance on detail-oriented tasks, while blue fosters creativity. Marketers use this knowledge to influence consumer behaviour, from packaging design to the look and feel of a website.

### How social proof influences our decisions

People tend to follow the actions of others, especially in uncertain situations. Because of this, social proof is another common tactic marketers use, often highlighting customer reviews, testimonials and the popularity of a product to create a sense of trust and reliability. When you see that others have had a positive experience with a product, your subconscious mind is more likely to follow suit, feeling reassured by the approval of the crowd.[9]

Another study found that hotel guests were more likely to reuse towels when informed that the majority of previous guests did the same.[10] This shows how powerful the influence of social proof can be in shaping behaviour and decisions.

## The impact of product placement

In the shops, strategic product placement is used to influence your buying choices. Products placed at eye level are more likely to be purchased because they are more noticeable. End-of-aisle displays and checkout counter placements are prime spots for impulse buys, often filled with high-profit, unhealthy snacks.

The supermarket layout itself is meticulously planned to maximise spending. Essentials like milk and bread are often located at the back of the store, forcing you to walk past numerous tempting products. Fresh produce is typically placed near the entrance to create a perception of healthiness and to stimulate your appetite, making you more likely to buy additional items.

## The lure of special offers

Then the use of scarcity and urgency in marketing can lead to impulsive purchases. Limited-time offers and flash sales create a fear of missing out (FOMO), compelling you to buy items you might not need or even want. This tactic taps into the primal part of your brain that reacts to perceived threats to resources, driving you to make irrational decisions.[11]

By understanding and countering the subtle influences of these marketing tactics, you can become more aware of how your environment is designed to influence your choices, take steps to counteract these effects, take back control of your food choices and make decisions that align with your health and wellness goals.

---

## How You Can Take Back Control

*Create a positive environment*

Surround yourself with visual and auditory cues that promote health and well-being. This could include displaying motivational quotes, keeping healthy foods visible and accessible, and listening to podcasts or music that uplift your mood and inspire healthy behaviours. The more you immerse yourself in positive stimuli, the more likely you are to make choices that align with your goals.

*Be mindful of the media*

Choose media that supports your health and well-being journey. Follow social media accounts that share healthy recipes, fitness tips and motivational content. Watch documentaries or read books that educate and inspire you about health and wellness.

By filling your media diet with positive primes, you reinforce your commitment to a healthy lifestyle.

---

## Go looking for support

Join groups or communities that share your health and wellness goals. Whether it's a local fitness class, an online support group or a healthy cooking club, engaging with like-minded individuals can provide powerful positive primes. These interactions not only offer support but also continually remind you of your objectives and inspire you to stay on track.

## Practise positive self-talk

Your internal dialogue can also serve as a powerful prime. Revisit Chapter 5 and practise affirmations and positive self-talk to reinforce your healthy intentions. Phrases like, 'I am capable of making healthy choices' or 'I am committed to my well-being' can prime your mind to stay focused and motivated.

The more you engage in positive self-talk, the more it becomes a natural part of your thinking process.

## Stay informed and aware

Being aware of how marketers use priming, colour psychology and social proof can help you recognise when these techniques are being used on you. Knowledge is power, and understanding these strategies can help you make more conscious choices.

## Stick to a shopping list

Plan your meals and snacks ahead of time and create a shopping list. Then stick to it! This reduces the likelihood of impulse buys and helps you stay focused on your health goals. Avoid shopping when you're hungry, as this can make you more susceptible to cravings and impulse purchases.

## Shop round the edges

Most supermarkets are designed with fresh, whole foods like fruits, vegetables, meats and dairy around the perimeter. By focusing your shopping on these areas and avoiding the inner aisles, where processed foods are typically placed, you can make healthier choices.

## Question every choice

When you feel the urge to buy something on impulse, take a moment to ask yourself why. Are you influenced by an advert you saw, the placement of the product or its packaging? Reflecting on your motivations can help you make more deliberate and healthier choices.

## CHAPTER 24

# Launch Your Brain's Goal-Seeking Missile

Of all the things I've discovered about the brain during my many years of studying neuroscience, the extraordinary reticular activating system probably surprised me the most. Let's call it the RAS (pronounced RAZ) for short.

The RAS is the most powerful tool there is for equipping you to change the way you behave and the way you feel. It will unlock your potential and guide you to reach your goals. And all this is achieved by a small bundle of nerves, no thicker than a pencil, that sits in your brainstem.

Every second, your brain is being fed billions of pieces of information from your senses – every sight, sound, smell, touch and taste.[1] That's a whole lot of stimulation and it's too much for the brain to handle without going into meltdown. So the RAS acts as a filter, deciding what data needs to get through and what can safely be ignored. It means you're fully aware of what really matters and oblivious to what doesn't, so you're able to focus on what's important to you. If your goal is to lead a healthier lifestyle that means you lose weight and keep it off, think how vital it is to programme your RAS to search out the things that will make your goal possible and filter out any stimulus that's not needed.

The thing about a stimulus is that your brain has become conditioned over time to react to it in a certain way. A simple example is how the smell of freshly baked bread can make you feel hungry. That automatic reaction is controlled within your all-powerful subconscious mind and happens without you thinking about it. It's why depriving yourself of food on a diet, which requires a conscious effort and willpower, seldom works in the long term. As we've seen, the subconscious always wins because it's nature's way of ensuring survival – it makes you eat and drink, it controls your heartbeat and your digestive system, it fires up hormones and it alerts you with instant reactions to perceived danger. The subconscious is also where self-limiting beliefs and emotions are stored, just waiting to be triggered.[2]

So, if you're a 'failed' dieter and think you'll never lose weight or you're an emotional eater who turns to cake to cheer yourself up or alleviate boredom, it's so important to reset your RAS.

But before looking at how to do this, there's something important to understand about how the RAS operates – it reinforces what's in your subconscious. It's an automatic process that doesn't make judgements and it can't separate good behaviour from bad behaviour. So, if your most predominant belief, based on years of unsuccessful diets, is 'I can never lose weight and keep it off', then guess what neural pathways have been built in your brain? Yes, pathways to future failure.

The RAS will assume that all you're interested in is eating too much so you don't lose weight – even though, at a logical level, you know full well that eating differently would help you lose weight. So it filters out all the helpful information and your brain only takes in the unhelpful stuff. Now, food will be everywhere you look. And because the RAS controls emotional responses, you'll find it impossible to resist temptations.

Suppose your belief, again based on years of negative experiences, is 'I hate exercise, it's a waste of time and effort', then the neural pathways will tell your RAS to make sure you never walk, jog or swim. Once again, the conscious part of your brain knows that more exercise can only be good for your health and your waistline. But the RAS will instinctively guide you to what it believes to be your goal – becoming an overweight couch potato. It's a goal that's all too easy to achieve in a culture like ours. But don't despair – you *can* do something about it.

You *can* retrain your RAS. You *can* create a healthier new you. And it's going to be a lot easier than you think because your RAS is very adaptable providing you feed it the right info. Let me show you.

Maybe you decided you would buy a new red car. Suddenly all you ever noticed was shiny red cars. Yellow ones, blue ones, white ones just seemed to fade into the background. This didn't happen by chance. Your positive thoughts about red cars had created new neural pathways and your RAS had sprung into action to filter out anything that wasn't about this new subject.

So if it's that easy to programme the RAS, it must be just as easy to reprogramme it to create change and start focusing your attention on healthy eating and exercise. The RAS loves goals. It feeds on them and propels you towards achieving them. Give it positive thoughts and it will create neural pathways that lead you towards positive outcomes. Once you feed it the right kind of information, it launches its own automatic guidance system and becomes a goal-seeking missile.

You have to tell it: 'I can lose weight and I will lose weight.' Tell it: 'I love exercise and I will do it three times a week.' Or even better, every day! That's how neural pathways and new behaviours are formed. Firstly, you set your goal and then you reinforce the intention by making sure your RAS is getting regular doses of positive data.

Change what you tell yourself! When you find yourself thinking about what you don't want, change it to what you *do* want. By restating negatives in the positive you'll reset your RAS filter so it switches to looking for uplifting experiences. Take the time to rewrite the negatives as the exact opposite. For example:

- 'I can't lose weight' becomes 'I can lose weight.'
- 'I can't stop snacking' becomes 'I can stop snacking.'
- 'I hate all exercise' becomes 'I love all exercise.'

Your RAS performs best with clear, precise guidance and writing it down really works. One study suggests that you are 42 per cent more likely to achieve your goals if you write them down, commit to action, have an accountability partner and share weekly progress reports with someone.[3]

So start the ball rolling by writing down your goals and keep your positives somewhere you can see them regularly. If your positive is 'I can stop snacking' then stick it on the fridge door. This constant positive reinforcement is crucial because habits are formed through repetition. The more times you see what you can do, the more times you will do it.[4]

## How You Can Take Back Control
### Visualise clear goals
Write down specific goals and visualise them regularly. Imagine your goals as already achieved, creating a vivid mental picture. This primes your RAS to recognise opportunities and resources that can help you achieve your goals.

### Use positive affirmations
In this way, you can programme your RAS to focus on your strengths and potential. Repeating affirmations like 'I can do this and it's working' or 'I can lose 0.5kg (1lb) a week' reinforces positive beliefs and intentions.

### Surround yourself with cues
Create an environment that supports your goals by surrounding yourself with visual and auditory reminders: inspirational notes on the fridge door, an uplifting ring tone on your phone, background music that aligns with your aspirations or favourite clothes hanging on the wardrobe door.

# CHAPTER 25

# Identify the 'Big Why' of Weight Loss

Setting goals can be daunting, especially if you've struggled to achieve them in the past and you have an innate fear of failure. But here's a comforting thought: goals are not about success or failure; they are about learning and adapting.

When you set a goal and don't quite reach it, it's not a failure. It's feedback – a chance to tweak your approach and move closer to success next time.

Various studies of the process of goal-setting have indicated that, if done correctly, it can help to make weight loss easier.[1] When you set clear, actionable goals, your brain becomes more focused, your motivation increases and the perception of difficulty diminishes.

An essential aspect of maintaining motivation is the desire for your goal. The more you want it, the less you'll be bothered by obstacles along the way. This phenomenon is supported by a study which found that motivation and physiological factors significantly influence how we perceive challenges.[2]

Identifying a compelling reason for your goal – what I call the Big Why – is crucial. Think deeply about why you want to achieve your goal. It has to evoke emotion and be meaningful to you. Whether it's fitting into a special dress for an event or improving your health after a doctor's warning, your Big Why will drive your momentum and motivation.

Visualise yourself at the end of your journey: wearing that dress, feeling healthier, playing energetically with your children or your grandchildren. This vivid mental image creates a strong connection with your goal. Your unconscious mind cannot distinguish between reality and imagination. By vividly imagining your end result, your mind starts to accept it as fact, making you more likely to achieve it. This concept is backed by research that explains how visualising your goals helps create new neural pathways that align with your desired behaviours (see the next chapter for more on visualisation).[3]

Another powerful technique is to identify fully with the person you will be once you've reached your goal. Transport yourself mentally to the future where you have already achieved your goal. Ask yourself: 'Who will I be when I'm in that outfit that's two sizes smaller? How will I behave? What will I eat? How will I feel?' By embodying the identity of your future self, you reinforce the behaviours and mindset needed to reach your goal.

Once you have a clear vision and a strong emotional connection to your goal, it's time to break it down into manageable pieces. This method, known as chunking down, is crucial because the brain prefers to aim at something that's not too far in the future. Setting smaller, short-term goals that lead up to your main goal helps maintain motivation and provides regular feedback on your progress.

For instance, if your goal is to fit into a swimsuit in three months, set weekly goals such as healthy eating targets or exercise milestones. Celebrating these small wins keeps you positive and motivated. Importantly, include small healthy rewards in your plan. If your brain knows there's a treat in the near future, cravings diminish. This approach is supported by research showing that setting specific, achievable goals and rewarding yourself for meeting them significantly enhances goal commitment and success.[4]

It's also beneficial to make your goals public. Sharing your goals with friends, family or an accountability partner can increase your commitment to achieving them, but be cautious about using social media as this can attract negative comments from strangers. Writing down your goals and displaying them in a visible place, such as on your bathroom mirror, reinforces your commitment and provides constant positive reinforcement.

When setting goals, it's essential to be specific. Vague goals like 'lose weight' are less effective than specific ones like 'lose ten pounds in three months by exercising three times a week and eating five servings of vegetables a day'. Specific goals provide clear direction and measurable outcomes, making it easier to track progress and make necessary adjustments.

Maintaining a positive internal dialogue is also crucial when it comes to realising your dreams. Replace negative thoughts like 'I can't do this' with positive affirmations like 'I am capable of achieving my goals.' This shift in mindset can significantly impact your motivation and resilience, and is supported by research that shows that people with a positive outlook are more likely to achieve their goals and feel satisfied with their progress.[5]

Understanding the neuroscience behind goal-setting can further enhance your efforts. As we saw earlier, the brain's reward system, primarily driven by dopamine, is activated when we set and achieve goals (see page 15). This activation creates feelings of pleasure and satisfaction, encouraging us to continue working towards our objectives.[6]

Remember, goal-setting is not just about reaching the destination; it's about enjoying the journey and learning from every step along the way.

## How You Can Take Back Control

*Define your Big Why*
Identify a compelling, emotional reason for your goal. This will keep you motivated and focused.

*Be specific and detailed*
Write down clear, specific goals with measurable outcomes. This clarity helps you track progress and make adjustments.

*Chunk down your goals*
Break your main goal into smaller, short-term targets. A lady on my Slimpod programme wanted to go from size 22 jeans to size 14 in 6 months. That's a lovely goal to work with so I suggested she start by making her first mini goal a size 20. When she was into her size 20s the next mini goal would be a size 18 and then, when she'd got into those, get the 16s out and so on. The goal each month was now much smaller and, to her unconscious mind, much more achievable.

So begin with a large final goal then work your way backwards and chunk it down so the goals on the way become much smaller. You'll know what your body is capable of so be realistic and you might get a lovely surprise. Remember to celebrate small wins to maintain motivation.

*Make your goals public*
Share your goals with others and display them in a visible place to reinforce commitment and accountability. I use Post-It notes on my laptop screen or the fridge door.

Next up, I want to share a top performance tip from professional sports stars that you can use every day to enhance your weight-loss success.

## Case Study: How I Took Back Control

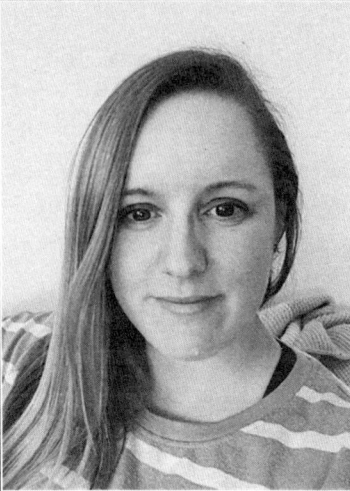

*Dr Victoria Baxter*

My earliest memory of food being a 'thing' was when I was a teenager. As soon as I started to earn my own money at 15, I would spend most of it on takeaways, reinforcing the idea of food as reward after a hard day at work. In adulthood, I struggled with yo-yo dieting. I used WeightWatchers to lose 20kg (3st), but it gradually crept back on over my thirties because, once I had a child, I couldn't keep up with the exercise routine that had helped me manage my weight until then.

I returned to WeightWatchers after maternity leave and was a pro by this point – I had learned to manipulate the 'points' system to 'allow' me to still enjoy the takeaways and wine I wanted at the weekend through near starvation during the week.

However, it was a moment one weekend in 2020, when I was getting annoyed trying to do the points 'maths' to allow me a kebab, that I realised I'd had enough. Someone said to me: 'Why are you bothering, you're only going to get the kebab anyway' and that hit the nail right on the head. The next day, I started to research nutrition and never looked back.

I've not dieted a day since. As I learned more about nutrition and a concept called intuitive eating, I realised that I needed to address my mindset and challenge myself on my food 'rules' (the main one being that a meal had to consist of three components) to make effective change. I encouraged myself to eat single bowls of wholesome and tasty foods for tea until it stopped feeling so 'wrong'.

I work as an NHS clinical psychologist and I started to 'practise what I preach' by using a psychological therapy called Acceptance and Commitment Therapy to help me work out what mattered most to me in life – what Sandra calls the 'Big Why'. I realised that my Big Why was being healthy for my daughter and, to achieve this, I had to build a new relationship with food.

While this began to help shift my relationship with food in a healthier direction, I had periods of time when old diet-mentality slipped back in and, by the time I found Slimpod in 2024, I hadn't lost any weight or inches. I was happier in feeling some freedom from dieting, but, for my health, I really did need to lose some weight.

Since joining Slimpod, I feel I've finally cracked it. It feels like the missing piece of the jigsaw for me. I now have an instinctive desire to try new foods, to only eat when hungry, to turn down free food (this being the biggest shock to me!) and I'm living by a new mantra of 'consistency is key'. With these changes at a subconscious level reinforcing my conscious desire to improve my health, I've now lost a few pounds, dropped a dress size and, at a recent health check, all my stats were looking great, with just one area to work on (cholesterol).

Furthermore I've vastly reduced my alcohol intake and am back into running again – the first time properly since pre-pregnancy. I feel positive for the future and excited to keep seeing these health improvements.

The 'thing that comes to mind to keep you going', as Sandra tells us, is always my daughter's face. I'm so pleased I found my Big Why and finally actually *feel* at peace around food.

*Find out more about Victoria's story here:*

## CHAPTER 26

# Picture Your Success: The Role of Visualisation

Our brains process a lot of information by collecting images and storing them away. It's one of the reasons we hear people saying, 'Picture this . . .' Some people are a lot more visual than others, but, for everyone, seeing a goal or an ambition as a picture can make success much more likely.[1]

If you've ever watched a rugby match on TV, you might have noticed that some of the top professionals do funny-looking things with their eyes before taking an important kick. They seem to be seeing the end result of the kick before they take it, with their eyes following a definite route from ball to goal and back again several times. This important technique is called visualisation and scientists and sports psychologists have proved that it works to give you a better chance of success.[2] A study of athletes who regularly practised visualisation showed improvements in their skills, confidence and overall performance.

This technique is not just for athletes or high achievers, though; anyone can harness the power of visualisation to make lasting changes in their life.[3] When you visualise, you are essentially training your brain to become more familiar with your goals, making them feel more attainable and real.

This is why you need to visualise the weight loss you're going to achieve. Seeing in your mind's eye the way your new shape will look at a future event – like a wedding, christening, party or on the beach – gives your unconscious mind a powerful target to aim at.

There are two types of visualisation – outcome and process – which work differently but which can be combined for the best possible results. Research supports both forms of visualisation, showing their effectiveness in achieving goals.[4]

**Outcome visualisation**

This involves imagining yourself achieving your goal. For the best results, create a vivid and colourful mental picture of the end result – include smells, tastes, touch as well as vision and sound. The more of your senses you use to create your image, the more effective it will be.

If you're visualising yourself looking slim at a special event, for example, go into real detail: where is it taking place, what precisely are you wearing, what size will your outfit be, who is there with you, who's making flattering comments about your new look, what are they saying and how does it feel?

**Process visualisation**

This involves imagining the steps needed to reach your goal. Instead of picturing yourself slimmer – the outcome – you visualise daily actions like choosing healthy foods and exercising. For example, see yourself preparing a nutritious breakfast each morning.

Visualising the process of healthy eating and regular exercise can help embed these behaviours into your routine, making it easier to stick to your goals. By mentally rehearsing positive actions, you prepare your mind and body to follow through with them in real life.[5]

Research shows that people who use visualisation experience significant improvements in their ability to adhere to exercise routines and achieve weight-loss goals. The study concludes that mental rehearsal can enhance self-efficacy and motivation, leading to better outcomes.[6]

Recent research using brain scans has shown that visualisation works because neurons in your brain, which uses minute electrical impulses to transmit information, can't tell the difference between an image you're imagining and a real-life action. When you visualise yourself doing something, the brain sends out an electrical impulse, which tells your neurons to perform the action. This in turn creates what's known as a new neural pathway, in effect a chain of brain cell clusters.[7]

By creating neural pathways related to weight loss and your behaviours around food, you can prime your body to act consistently and precisely in the way you've imagined – eating more healthily so you lose weight.

Here's how visualisation works for weight loss:

• **Enhances motivation:** Visualising your ideal self can create a powerful sense of motivation. By imagining the benefits of reaching your weight-loss goals, such as improved health, increased energy and enhanced self-esteem, you can boost your determination to stick to your plan.

- **Builds confidence:** Seeing yourself successfully following a healthy lifestyle can build confidence in your ability to achieve your goals. This mental rehearsal prepares your mind for the challenges ahead, making you more resilient when faced with obstacles.
- **Fosters a positive mindset:** Visualisation can counteract negative self-talk and self-doubt. By focusing on positive outcomes and visualising success, you can shift your mindset from one of scarcity and fear to one of abundance and possibility.
- **Creates a clear plan:** Visualisation helps you develop a clear, detailed plan for achieving your goals. By mentally rehearsing the steps you need to take, you can increase your awareness of potential obstacles and identify strategies to overcome them.

Visualisation is not a substitute for action – nothing is – but it's a valuable complement to it. You must combine your mental imagery with practical steps towards your goals. If you visualise yourself eating healthy meals, then plan and prepare nutritious foods to reinforce this image. This consistent practice of visualisation and action creates a powerful synergy, driving you closer to your weight-loss goals.

Visualisation can also help you build resilience and overcome challenges. By mentally rehearsing how you will handle setbacks and obstacles, you can prepare yourself to respond with confidence and determination. Mental preparation can reduce anxiety and increase your ability to stay focused on your goals, even when faced with difficulties.

The benefits of visualisation extend beyond weight loss.

This technique can be applied to various aspects of life, including career advancement, personal relationships and overall well-being. By visualising success in different areas, you can enhance your confidence, motivation and resilience, leading to a more fulfilling and balanced life.

Remember, the key is consistency, specificity and combining mental rehearsal with action. Set aside time each day to visualise your success, engage all your senses and use your mental images to guide your behaviour.

With practice and persistence, you can harness the power of visualisation to achieve your weight-loss goals and create a more fulfilling life.

**A free gift for you: Sample my Mind Magic**

Experience the power of the mind–body connection with a free practical tool you can download from my website. Just scan this QR code with your phone:

It will give you exclusive access to a remarkable recording called 'The Power Shower', which you can listen to any time you need to de-stress and relax after a hard day. The Power Shower is the ultimate visualisation exercise and guides your mind to wash away what I call 'the dirt of the day' in a matter of minutes. Whenever I listen to the calming male voice it leaves me feeling calm, refreshed and relaxed. Now that's Mind Magic!

---

### How You Can Take Back Control

*Be specific*

When visualising your goals, be as specific as possible. Imagine each step you will take, such as choosing healthy foods and exercising regularly. Specific visualisation makes your goals more tangible and achievable.

*Engage all your senses*

Make your visualisation vivid by incorporating all your senses. Picture the sights, sounds, smells, tastes and feelings associated with your success. This sensory detail enhances the effectiveness of your mental imagery.

*Practise regularly*

Consistency is crucial for successful visualisation. Dedicate a few minutes each day, either in the morning to set a positive tone or in the evening to reinforce your goals. Regular practice strengthens the neural pathways.

*Combine with action*

Plan and prepare for the actions you visualise, such as cooking healthy meals or scheduling workouts. Combining mental rehearsal with practical steps maximises your chances of success.

---

Next, the big question: are you in control of your life or is life in control of you? I'll show you how to be Master of Your Life.

# CHAPTER 27

# Become the Internal Master of Your Life

When I learned about the psychological concept of 'locus of control', it changed my life, and now when I discuss the subject in my Zooms or live chats, it fascinates members of my Slimpod programme and has a huge impact on many of them, too.

Locus of control refers to the degree to which individuals believe they have control over the events that affect their lives. This concept, introduced in the 1950s, can be broadly divided into two categories: internal and external.[1]

Individuals with an external locus of control (EXLOC) feel their lives are controlled by external forces, such as luck, fate, other people or events. They often believe they have little influence over what happens to them and that their efforts don't significantly impact their outcomes. It's when we think our lives are shaped by things outside of us, that the world has the power to make us feel things.

Conversely, people with an internal locus of control (ILOC) believe they are the masters of their fate. They attribute their successes and failures to their own actions, decisions and efforts. They tend to take responsibility for their lives and believe their hard work, choices and personal qualities determine their outcomes.

Understanding the difference between an ILOC and an EXLOC can empower you to take charge of your life and shape your destiny more effectively. This is especially crucial when it comes to managing your health and weight, where your beliefs about control can significantly impact your success.

An ILOC is often associated with positive psychological outcomes. People with this mindset are more likely to exhibit resilience, take initiative, experience higher self-esteem and practise better self-regulation.[2]

They tend to recover quickly from setbacks because they believe they have the power to change their situation. They are proactive in pursuing their goals and solving problems, leading to greater personal and professional achievements.

They feel more confident in their abilities, which enhances their self-worth. They are more likely to engage in healthy behaviours and avoid negative ones, as they feel responsible for their well-being.[3]

An EXLOC, on the other hand, can lead to less favourable psychological outcomes in which people are more likely to feel helpless, experience anxiety and depression, lack motivation and engage in unhealthy behaviours.

They may develop a sense of helplessness and passivity, believing that their efforts are futile. The belief that they cannot control their lives can lead to heightened stress, anxiety and depression.

They may struggle to find the motivation to pursue their goals, as they believe their efforts will not make a difference.

They might be less likely to take care of their health and well-being, feeling that external factors determine their fate.[4]

Dieting often exacerbates an EXLOC. Many diet plans promise quick fixes and miraculous results, implying that success depends on the diet itself rather than the individual's efforts. This can lead to a sense of dependency on external factors and a feeling of powerlessness when the diet inevitably fails. Most people I speak to on my Slimpod programme feel they're stuck. When they start revealing their story, it's usually all about repeating things that just haven't worked for them. Usually diets, but other patterns emerge, too. The constant cycle of dieting and failing can reinforce the belief that weight loss is beyond your control, further entrenching an EXLOC.[5]

Taking responsibility for what happens to you is the difference between saying: 'I'm a failure because all those diets have never worked for me' and: 'Sod the diet, I'm going to take control and make this happen.'

In my experience, people with an ILOC are generally happier and more successful in their personal and professional lives. They are better at coping with stress and have a greater sense of satisfaction and well-being. An ILOC mindset puts you back in the driving seat. Remember: nobody can take your power; you can only give it away.

If you recognise that you have an EXLOC, don't despair. You can cultivate a more internal locus with conscious effort and practice. In any situation where you have a choice or where life is throwing a spanner in the works, start learning to ask yourself, 'What is it I can do here?' This will open up your mind to possibility. Life will always throw obstacles in your path; it's the way you respond to these obstacles that makes the difference. It's about taking ACTION! There's nearly always something you can do and anything more than nothing is something.

---

### How You Can Take Back Control

*Recognise your power*

Acknowledge you have the power to influence your life. Identify areas where you can make changes and take small steps to assert control. Celebrate these small victories to build your confidence and reinforce your belief in your ability to shape your destiny.

*Set realistic goals*

Set achievable goals that are within your control. Break larger goals into smaller, manageable tasks, and focus on what you can do to achieve them. This approach helps you see the direct impact of your actions and enhances your sense of control.

*Think what's possible*

If you feel you've run into a dead end and nothing's working, don't give up. Start asking yourself, 'What is it I can do here?' Open up your mind to possibility and be positive: 'I can find a way.'

---

## Case Study: How I Took Back Control

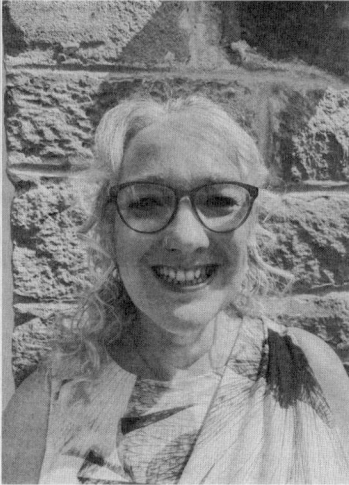

*June Ward*

I had a choice: let my chronic illness take over my life or take control and be me. I chose to be me. I refused to be defined by fibromyalgia, which had put me in a mobility scooter and on crutches. For too many years, it controlled me.

I couldn't walk without pain and was essentially housebound. I relied on my elderly parents to take me into town for groceries. My 76-year-old dad would carry my shopping because I didn't have the energy to do it myself. It was humiliating, but I was so grateful for their help.

I was pensioned off from the NHS before I turned 40, and my world felt so small. Then I joined Slimpod four years ago and that was the best decision of my life. It made me believe that I could be free of the body I had been living in and that I had the power to change it. The energy I gained gave me the motivation to move more. I learned to appreciate my body, to be patient with myself and to understand that slow and steady progress paid off.

I've tackled treetop walks in Wales, zip lines, and joined a gym. I've lost 25.5kg (4st), dropping from a size 20 to a 14. But, more importantly, I'm free. I've become a confident and empowered woman who no longer feels guilty about food or drink, although I naturally drink far less than I used to.

I no longer need antidepressants because I'm not depressed anymore. I feel like a completely different person on a new path. Even my painkillers have become less necessary as my increased activity improves my symptoms.

Fibro no longer rules me – I am in charge of it. I've become a natural eater, no longer ruled by diet books, scales or food, and I can even say no to my mum's offers of second helpings.

When I started Slimpod, I couldn't even stand on one leg. Now, I can stand on one leg on top of a chair. I am a completely different woman – confident, independent and purposeful. I'm so happy now, I take too many selfies! I love myself and my body.

I've forgiven myself for feeling fat and thanked my body for giving me two amazing boys. My body has fought its battles, and I keep going. I even have a boudoir photo wall in my bedroom, and my proudest photo is the one in my burlesque red basque.

*Find out more about June's story here:*

## CHAPTER 28

# Be a 'Can Do' Person: The Power of Belief

Over the past 15 years, one of the biggest things I've noticed about people who come on my Slimpod programme with a history of yo-yo dieting is that they've stopped believing anyone or anything can help them lose weight. They've given up believing it's even possible. So many also have the belief that they're failures, and it's a dreadful combination. But it *can* be changed!

Henry Ford once said: 'Whether you think you can, or you think you can't – you're right.' This is what he was driving at: believing you can't do something is a self-fulfilling prophecy. Tell yourself you can't lose weight, and you'll fail. But tell yourself you can and then really believe in yourself, and everything changes. I constantly tell people on my Facebook Lives that the most important step to changing something in your life is to believe you can do it.

It's really easy to understand why your self-belief won't be high if you've been beaten down mentally by constantly losing three stone then ending up putting it back on (and more) over and over again. Your brain has been programmed by past experiences to believe that you can't lose weight, and that becomes a terrible self-limiting belief. If you don't believe you can succeed, why would you even try?

You need to know that your brain is wrong. You *can* cultivate self-belief and you *can* achieve things. Seeing that change of attitude in people over the years is one of the things that gives me the most pleasure. Because when you start believing you can, it's the foundation of success, empowerment and happiness.

Self-belief is more than just optimism; it's the conviction that you can exert control over your own motivation, behaviour and social environment. Too many people don't believe that's possible, so I'm going to share the science that proves that it works.

There are two parts to believing in yourself and it's useful to understand the difference – and how it's possible for one to be high while the other is low. It explains why so many people are baffled by the fact that they have the confidence to be successful at work, the arts or leisure activities, but when it comes to losing weight they don't believe in themselves to ever succeed.

In psychology, self-efficacy and self-belief are related concepts, but they are not exactly the same:

- Self-efficacy refers to your belief in your ability to perform specific tasks or achieve specific goals. It means you can have high self-efficacy in one area (for example, academic performance) and low self-efficacy in another (for example, sports).
- Self-belief, on the other hand, is a broader term that encompasses your overall confidence and belief in your

abilities and potential. It includes self-efficacy, but also extends to a general sense of self-worth and the belief that you can handle life's challenges and achieve your broader goals.

Both influence how you think, feel and act, and both are crucial for achieving personal success and maintaining motivation – but they operate at different levels of specificity.

According to psychologist Albert Bandura, who first introduced the concept, high self-efficacy means having the confidence to take on challenges, recover quickly from setbacks and remain committed to goals despite obstacles.[1] Low self-belief, on the other hand, can lead to avoidance of challenging tasks, giving up easily and a tendency to see difficulties as threats rather than opportunities.

Let's consider what this means to you: which elements below sound very familiar?

## If you have high self-efficacy

- **You relish a challenge:** You view difficult tasks as goals to be mastered rather than threats to be avoided. You are more likely to embrace challenges and persist in the face of setbacks.[2]
- **You're emotionally stable:** You're more resilient and can manage stress better than others. The belief in your abilities provides a buffer against anxiety and depression.[3]
- **You set yourself goals:** You always set realistic yet challenging goals and are committed to achieving them. You're proactive in your efforts and find satisfaction in your progress.[4]

## If you have low self-efficacy

- **You avoid challenges:** You tend to avoid difficult tasks and are more likely to give up when faced with obstacles. You often see challenges as insurmountable barriers.[5]
- **You're emotionally vulnerable:** You're more susceptible to stress and anxiety, often feeling overwhelmed by your perceived inability to effect change.[6]
- **You set lower goals:** You set lower goals or avoid setting them altogether, doubting your capacity to achieve them. This lack of direction can lead to a sense of stagnation and helplessness.[7]

So, what impact does self-belief have on your goal of sustainable weight loss?

## If you believe you can't

- **You self-sabotage:** Negative self-belief can mean you skip workouts or indulge in unhealthy foods. This mindset creates a self-fulfilling prophecy where the expectation of failure leads to actions that ensure it.[8]
- **You lack motivation:** Believing that you can't succeed diminishes your motivation to try. This often results in half-hearted efforts and a quick return to old habits.[9]
- **Your stress increases:** The stress of feeling inadequate can lead to emotional eating and other behaviours that counteract weight-loss efforts. This cycle can be difficult to break and often leads to frustration and defeat.[10]

## If you believe you can

- **You never give up:** A strong belief in your ability to succeed fosters resilience. You're more likely to push through tough times and stay committed to your goals.[11]
- **You're proactive:** Self-belief encourages proactive behaviours. You're more likely to plan meals, stick to exercise routines and seek out support when needed.[12]
- **You're super-positive:** Each success, no matter how small, reinforces your belief in your ability to succeed. This creates a positive feedback loop where confidence breeds more success.[13]

Losing weight is as much a mental challenge as a physical one. Believing in your ability to succeed is not just a motivational phrase; it's a psychological necessity. Self-belief empowers you to take control of your actions and keep going through challenges. It transforms obstacles into opportunities and setbacks into lessons.

And **you can do this**, even if you haven't really believed you can do it before; even if you've tried and not succeeded. Each time something doesn't work, your brain learns it doesn't work. But how about this – what if you didn't have such a fixed belief that it doesn't work and started thinking there's possibly a different way to tackle the problem? Open up your mind to possibility and the idea of winning!

## How You Can Take Back Control

*Set small, achievable goals*

Start with manageable goals to build confidence. Each small victory will reinforce your belief in your ability to succeed. For instance, aim to drink more water daily or add an extra ten minutes to your exercise routine.[14]

*Visualise success*

Use the power of visualisation to see yourself achieving your weight-loss goals (see Chapter 26). Picture the steps you'll take and the results you'll achieve. This mental rehearsal can increase confidence and motivation.[15] But not everyone is able to visualise so, if that's you, it's not a deal breaker. You can still succeed!

*Celebrate progress*

Recognise and enjoy your progress, no matter how small. Each step forward is a victory and a testament to your ability to succeed. Keep a journal of your achievements and refer back to it when you need a confidence boost.[16]

The next chapter is all about how to develop a growth mindset. I know you'll enjoy it!

## Case Study: How I Took Back Control

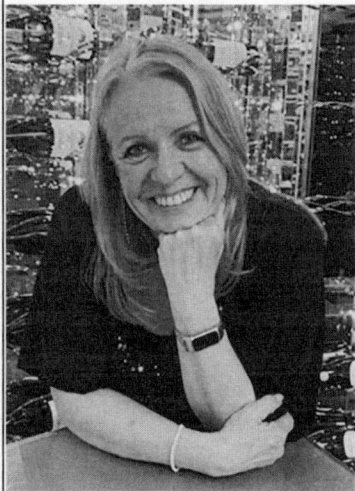

*Tanya Wakeford*

Like many others, I was overwhelmed by life's demands: eating too much, drinking too much and neglecting myself while caring for everyone else. As a mum of four with elderly parents, I was the main carer and worked full-time. My own well-being was always last on the list and, as a result, my health and weight spiralled out of control.

Over the years, I tried everything. I meticulously weighed and measured every bite, obsessed over the scales and still found myself stuck in the same cycle. It always felt like I was failing, and I would eventually give up, thinking I was destined to be overweight forever.

Life took a harder turn when my marriage failed. My husband, who had been my partner since I was 13, struggled with alcoholism. Despite our deep love for each other, his addiction became a battle I couldn't fight for him. We separated after nearly 38 years together and, though it was heartbreaking, it was necessary.

Then, I suffered a series of blows. My eldest brother died of cancer, then the following year my estranged husband died from a heart attack. Finally, my mum passed away after a stroke. I was barely holding on, trying to keep going for the sake of everyone else. My mind was a mess, and my health was slipping further away.

At my lowest point, I realised that, at 60, I was at the age when health problems could become life-threatening. I knew that if I didn't make a change, I might be next. That's when I came across Slimpod, which spoke to me in a way nothing else had.

The journey hasn't been easy, and it's far from over, but the difference now is that I feel empowered. My mindset has shifted – I'm not just focused on losing weight but on living a happier, healthier life. I'm taking care of myself in ways I never did before, and it's changing everything.

Now, I have the confidence to do things I never would have before. I even did my daily exercise session on the beach the other day. I've stopped saving clothes for 'special occasions'. Every day is a special occasion now because I'm here to live it. I recently wore a dress I had saved for two years and a woman stopped me to say she loved it! I also braved a bikini at the beach for the first time in 28 years. It was nerve-wracking, but I did it. The last time I wore one, I had a pregnancy bump and was proud of it. This time, I was proud of the progress I've made and the confidence I've gained.

Before, I hid from cameras and hated having photos taken. Now, I'm proud of my body. I even did a photo shoot last week – a whole day devoted to me! It was so much fun, and I loved it. Who is this person?

I'm not a new person; I'm just more of who I'm meant to be. I'm not Tanya doing something to please everybody else. I'm Tanya being Tanya. I put myself first now because if I'm not at my best, I can't give my best to others. I still care for everyone, but I've learned that I have to take care of myself first. It's not selfish; it's necessary.

*Find out more about Tanya's story here:*

## CHAPTER 29

# Harness the Power of a Growth Mindset

Do you think you can change? It's a question that might make you stop and ponder! The answer could be tied to whether you have a fixed or a growth mindset. The mindset concept is a psychological theory developed by Carol Dweck in her best-selling book *Mindset*, and it provides profound insight into how our beliefs about our abilities influence our behaviour and success.[1]

I've seen this reveal itself so much in people's weight-loss journeys. Over the years, I've encountered two sets of people on my Slimpod programme: those with a growth mindset who start with an attitude that they want to believe things can change, and others with a fixed mindset who have deeply ingrained beliefs that nothing works for them anymore. This often becomes a protection against failure.

I love seeing both sets of people develop and grow into the best version of themselves, but what exactly is the difference and which mindset do you have?

## A fixed mindset

People with a fixed mindset assume that their capacities – like their ability to lose weight or change their eating habits – are inherently static. They tend to avoid challenges, give up easily and see effort as fruitless. In the context of weight loss, this can manifest as a reluctance to try new healthier systems or exercise routines because of past failures.

If you have a fixed mindset, you might find yourself thinking, 'I can't stick to a diet' or 'I'm just not cut out for exercise' or 'I'm always going to be overweight because it's in my genes' or 'I've tried and failed before, so why bother?'

This mindset can lead to a sense of hopelessness and a self-fulfilling prophecy of failure, making sustainable weight loss seem unattainable. It can lead to a vicious cycle where fear of failure prevents you from taking the necessary steps towards your goals.

## A growth mindset

Those with a growth mindset thrive on challenge and see failures not as evidence of low intelligence or inability, but as a springboard for growth and for stretching their existing abilities. From this perspective, every challenge is an opportunity to learn, and every setback is a chance to adjust and persevere, fostering resilience and persistence.

For those seeking to lose weight, adopting a growth mindset means viewing each day as a new opportunity to improve your health and move closer to your goals. You see what's possible beyond your current abilities.

You are more likely to experiment with different weight-loss strategies, learn from your experiences and keep pushing forward despite difficulties. This positive outlook not only enhances motivation but also leads to more sustainable weight loss.

## Embracing a Growth Mindset

Having a growth mindset for weight loss is about making a fundamental shift from focusing on proving yourself to the scales to improving yourself. This mental transition is not just about losing weight – it's about learning, growing and ultimately thriving.

By believing in your capacity to change and embracing the journey's ups and downs, you unlock your true potential for success. Remember, it's a journey, not a destination. Each step you take towards embracing a growth mindset is a step towards a more empowered and fulfilling life.

When we delve into the research behind the growth mindset, we find compelling evidence that supports its benefits. Carol Dweck's pioneering work has shown that individuals with a growth mindset are more likely to embrace challenges, persist through obstacles and view effort as a pathway to mastery. This mindset fosters resilience and long-term achievement, both crucial for sustainable weight loss.

Another study found that employees with a growth mindset were more adaptable to change and performed better in dynamic work environments.[2] This adaptability can be directly applied to weight loss, where flexibility and resilience are key to overcoming the inevitable ups and downs.

Research also shows that a growth mindset can signifi-cantly reduce stress and anxiety, common barriers to success-ful weight management.[3] By viewing setbacks as opportuni-ties to learn rather than as failures, you can maintain a healthier mental state, which supports your physical health goals.

One study found that people with a growth mindset were more likely to engage in healthy behaviours, such as regular exercise and balanced nutrition.[4] This proactive approach to health is essential for lasting weight loss and overall well-being.

Finally, there is clear evidence that a growth mindset can enhance self-regulation, enabling people to stick to their health goals more effectively.[5] This self-discipline is vital for managing weight over the long term, as it helps you to navi-gate temptations and maintain healthy habits.

These research-backed insights show that developing a growth mindset is not just a theoretical concept, but a practi-cal tool for achieving lasting weight loss. It's about shifting your perspective, embracing the process and believing in your ability to change and grow.

## How You Can Take Back Control

*Set learning goals*

Instead of focusing solely on outcome goals, like losing a specific amount of weight, set learning goals that enhance your journey. For instance, aim to cook a new healthy recipe each week or understand more about the nutritional value of food. This approach emphasises skill development and understanding, which are key for long-term changes. As Carol Dweck points out: 'The view you adopt for yourself profoundly affects the way you lead your life.'[6]

*Embrace challenges*

When faced with difficult situations, such as resisting temptation at a party or pushing through a tough workout, see them as opportunities to grow stronger both mentally and physically. Challenges help you discover your real potential. Embracing these moments with a growth mindset can transform obstacles into stepping stones.[7]

*Celebrate efforts, not just results*

Recognise and reward yourself for the efforts you make, not just the pounds you lose. This could include applauding yourself for choosing healthy meals, exercising regularly or simply making better choices. Celebrating efforts reinforces the process of growth and learning, which is crucial for maintaining motivation.[8]

*Learn from setbacks*

Rather than beating yourself up over a small blip, analyse what led to it and how you can prevent similar situations in the future. Understanding that setbacks are part of the journey and learning from them is crucial. It's no good sitting back on your laurels and refusing to make further progress.

*Actively seek feedback*

Constructive criticism can be very valuable. Whether it's from a coach, a nutritionist or a supportive community, gaining insights from others can help you see progress and areas needing improvement that you might not notice on your own. Seeking feedback shows a willingness to learn and improve – key components of a growth mindset.[9]

One thing that will really help with developing a growth mindset, as we'll explore in the next chapter, is learning to be kinder to yourself. I call it 'loving yourself slimmer!'

# Case Study: How I Took Back Control

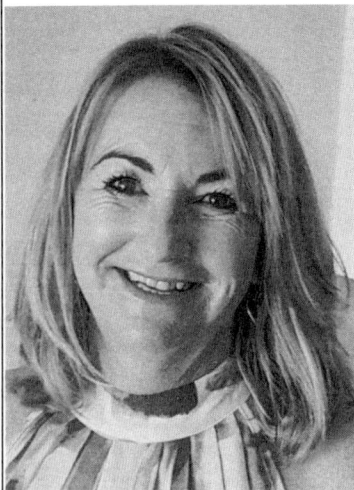

*Jane Harman*

I used to eat just about anything and everything. It didn't matter if I was full or even felt sick; I would keep eating until every last bit was gone. I couldn't resist food. I remember looking at my husband's plate and, if he left anything, I'd ask, 'Are you not going to eat that?' Then I'd finish it off without hesitation.

About five years ago, I was put on statins for my cholesterol, but I never really thought much about how I was living my life. I never thought I'd be able to change.

For a long time, I didn't understand myself or realise what was possible with the right growth mindset. I was stuck in self-limiting beliefs, falling into the same traps repeatedly, whether it was with dieting, relationships or just life in general.

But things started to change after I began the Slimpod programme. My eating and exercise habits transformed completely, along with my health. Slimpod taught me so much about the importance of whole foods and the dangers of ultra-processed foods. Now, I make better food choices effortlessly, without needing willpower.

The last three months have been incredible. I've lost

weight, which was my initial goal, but I've also gained a wealth of knowledge that's opened doors to better health and nutrition. Today, I found out that my cholesterol levels have improved so much that I can stop taking statins. I feel inspired by the changes I've made.

For over a year, I struggled with a hip and thigh problem that no doctor could diagnose. I underwent MRI scans, X-rays, ultrasounds, various physiotherapies and consulted two different traumatologists – all with no answers. As I read more about menopause, I realised that I didn't have to simply put up with the symptoms. I began to suspect that my joint pain was menopause-related.

Two weeks ago, I started HRT, and the difference is astounding. My hip no longer wakes me up at night, I can play golf without needing ibuprofen, and I no longer get up from a chair like an old woman. If it weren't for Slimpod, I never would have considered menopause as a factor.

Now, I'm two stone lighter and feel more in control of my emotions. I'm 57 years old, but I've never felt better. I've started weight training every other day and regularly go walking and swimming. I'm even thinking about becoming a menopause coach because of everything I've learned.

Looking back, I can hardly believe how much my life and my mindset have changed. It's not just about the weight loss, although that's been amazing. It's about gaining control, confidence and a renewed sense of joy.

The journey I've been on has made me happier, healthier and more positive than I ever thought possible.

*Find out more about Jane's story here:*

## CHAPTER 30

# Love Yourself Slimmer: The Science of Self-Compassion

When it comes to weight loss, many of us are our own worst critics. We berate ourselves for our slip-ups, compare our progress to others and often hold ourselves to impossible standards. I see it every day of the week in our Slimpod private group.

However, for lasting weight loss, it's vital that we harness the power of self-love.

Self-compassion is not just a feel-good concept – it is vital for boosting self-esteem and involves treating yourself with the same kindness and understanding you would offer to a friend. It means recognising that everyone makes mistakes and experiences setbacks, and it involves being patient and gentle with yourself during these times.

Self-compassion has been shown to have profound effects on both mental and physical health, and I witness this happening every single day in our community. It's the part of a person's transformation that I love the most!

One of the key reasons it is so powerful is that it helps to reduce stress. When you are kinder to yourself, you lower your levels of cortisol, the stress hormone. High levels of cortisol are linked to weight gain, particularly around the abdomen, because the body holds on to fat as a defence mechanism during times of stress.

A study by Dr Kristin Neff, a leading researcher in the field of self-compassion, found that individuals who practised self-compassion had lower levels of cortisol and higher levels of heart rate variability, which is a measure of how well the body can manage stress.[1]

Self-compassion also encourages a more balanced and less restrictive approach to eating. Dieting often involves strict rules, which can lead to a cycle of deprivation and bingeing. By contrast, being kind to yourself allows you to make healthier food choices without the associated guilt and shame when you occasionally indulge. Research has shown that mindfulness-based interventions, which include components of self-compassion, can significantly reduce binge eating and emotional eating.[2]

Here's another plus: self-compassion fosters resilience. When you treat yourself kindly, you are more likely to pick yourself up after a setback and continue striving towards your goals. This resilience is crucial for long-term weight loss, as the journey is rarely a smooth one.

I was fascinated by research which found that people who practised self-compassion were more likely to persevere after experiencing failure and were less likely to engage in negative self-talk.[3]

Another benefit of self-compassion is that it promotes a healthier body image. Many people struggling with weight issues have a negative perception of their bodies, which can lead to a host of psychological issues, including depression and anxiety. By practising self-compassion, you can improve your body image and overall mental health. Research has shown that treating yourself more kindly can lead to significant improvements in body image and reductions in body shame.[4]

It can also enhance motivation and self-discipline. While it might seem counter-intuitive, being kind to yourself can actually help you stick to your goals more effectively than being self-critical. When you approach your weight-loss journey with self-compassion, you are more likely to set realistic goals and create sustainable habits.

One study found that self-compassionate people were more likely to engage in healthy behaviours, such as regular exercise and balanced eating, because they were motivated by a desire to care for themselves rather than a fear of failure.[5]

One final thing: being nice to yourself can also help you build a supportive internal dialogue. Instead of the inner critic that we met in Chapter 17, who constantly undermines your efforts, you develop an inner coach who encourages and uplifts you. This positive internal dialogue is essential for maintaining motivation and self-esteem throughout your weight-loss journey.

It's important to note that self-compassion is not about letting yourself off the hook or avoiding responsibility. Rather, it involves acknowledging your imperfections and committing to self-improvement in a kind and understanding way. It's about finding a balance between accepting yourself as you are and striving to be the best version of yourself.

So how can you start practising this today? One simple way is to become more mindful of your self-talk. Pay attention to the way you speak to yourself, especially during challenging times. If you notice negative or critical thoughts, try to reframe them in a more compassionate way. For example, instead of saying, 'I can't believe I messed up again', try saying, 'It's okay to make mistakes. I'm learning and growing every day.'

Another effective technique is to treat yourself with the same kindness and understanding you would offer to a friend. When you're feeling down or frustrated, imagine what you would say to a loved one in the same situation, and then say those words to yourself.

Being grateful for what you've got, instead of moaning about what you haven't got, can also help you to cultivate a more compassionate mindset. Take time each day to reflect on the things you appreciate about yourself and your life. Maybe even text yourself a special note of something really special now and again. This can help shift your focus away from your perceived flaws and towards your strengths and achievements.

Engaging in self-care activities is also important. Make time for activities that bring you joy and relaxation, whether that's taking a walk in nature, reading a good book or spending time with loved ones. By taking care of your mental and physical well-being, you reinforce the message to yourself that you are worthy of love and care.

Finally, remember that this is a skill that takes time and practice to develop. Be patient with yourself and recognise that it's okay to have setbacks. The important thing is to keep trying and to treat yourself with kindness and understanding along the way.

The science is clear: self-compassion is not just a feel-good concept, but a vital component of successful weight loss. So go ahead and give yourself the love and compassion you deserve – your mind and body will thank you for it.

### How You Can Take Back Control

*Mind your self-talk*

Revisit Chapter 5 and pay attention to how you speak to yourself, especially in challenging times. Replace negative thoughts with compassionate and encouraging ones.

*Treat yourself like a friend*

When you're feeling down, imagine what you would say to a loved one in the same situation and say those words to yourself.

*Practise gratitude*

Reflect on the things you appreciate about yourself and your life each day. This can help shift your focus from flaws to strengths.

*Engage in self-care*

Make time for activities that bring you joy and relaxation, reinforcing the message that you are worthy of love and care. Because you are!

## Case Study: How I Took Back Control

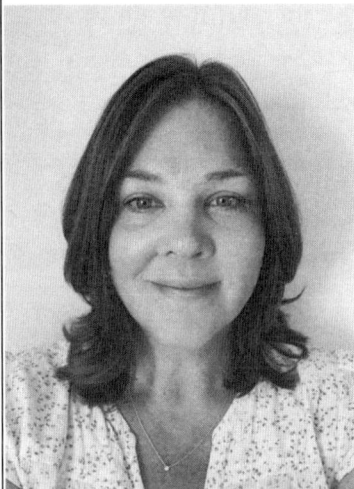

*Poppy Hinton*

For ten years, I'd had a conversation rattling round in my head. It was with a lovely young lady who'd had children and put on weight, but she was so contented with the way she was in life that she didn't even care about losing weight or not. I thought at the time, 'My God, that's amazing, you're thinking about loving yourself as you are.' Ever since, I've been trying to decide if could love this person that I was.

My size had really crept up, despite trying to lose weight by dieting, and Covid was a challenging time for me. I vowed 100 per cent that I was not dying on a diet and that's when I went full-on – 'let's eat everything in the world'. Before I knew it I was a size 24 and I was tired and feeling sorry for myself. I'd stand in front of the mirror in horrible clothes looking miserable.

On New Year's Day three years ago I decided that I wanted to be happy again. I started looking for something that would change my mindset and discovered Slimpod. I can hardly believe the changes it has helped me to achieve. The first thing I noticed was that I stopped snacking and eating in between meals. It happened like magic.

Suddenly, instead of eating a whole box of sweet grapes, I'd put some in a small bowl and that would be enough to satisfy me. Being aware of those kinds of habits is definitely the first step to conquering them. I've gone off bread completely, especially shop-bought sandwiches because they all seem so boring now. I prefer a salad. I'll never have a burger and chips again – not because I can't, but because I don't want them. And I constantly look at other people's meals and think, 'that's far too much food'.

Being positive about my day is a big cue for happiness. If I feel I've had a bit of a wobbly time, rather than go and eat something I think, 'Right, I'm just gonna write down all the positive things about my day and focus on that.' Previously, when something upset me it would definitely have driven me to food.

Today, I'm a size 14. And I now have the confidence and desire to celebrate things with a big party. I can wear something a little bit tighter. I accept, share and embrace how I look and feel, enjoying every moment.

I even committed to an exercise challenge to raise money for a charity, something I never ever would have done before. I was so excited, scared and ready to have a go – and I did it. I ran 100k (62 miles) before my fiftieth birthday and, for me, that was a win, win, win!

Now I've lost so much weight, but, importantly, I've got my shine back and more. I'm braver, I'm more confident (in a way I didn't know I needed), I love life more, I manage my anxiety differently, I'll have a go, move out of my comfort zone and really feel proud of myself. My default is happy and positive.

Slimpod has changed my perception of myself. I went roller skating with my daughter this weekend, which I never would have done when I was a size 24. I'd have been too embarrassed to get out there: 'What if I fell, how would they get me back up? People might look at me.' After all this time, I'm still having fun discovering the new me.

*Find out more about Poppy's story here:*

## CHAPTER 31

# Liberate Yourself With Healthy Eating

There's so much confusion about healthy eating and dieting, and yet they're very different. Be careful not to confuse dieting with diet. Your diet is about the food you eat every day to keep you healthy. For example, my diet consists of about 80 per cent healthy food and 20 per cent not so healthy, but that's the balance of a normal diet or a normal eater.

When you've been dieting, calorie counting or following food plans for years, you become conditioned to eating food purely to make the scales move. The focus isn't on nourishing and fuelling your body so that it operates at its best, both mentally and physically. Yet, where weight loss is concerned, the outcomes are often the same.

In my Slimpod community, food, diet, dieting and healthy eating come up a lot because my programme doesn't have a food plan, and people struggle with the idea of not following some sort of structured plan. People often think: 'What is this – no food plan to follow? How can that work?'

But the aim is to become a normal eater. Until about 60 years ago, there were no diets or food plans. There was also no obesity crisis. Do you think these factors could be related?

A lot of people, even unconsciously, revert to dieting when they start my programme and then wonder why they feel like they're falling off the wagon after about three weeks. They haven't allowed the Slimpod time to work its magic because they're still in conscious control of what they're eating – out of pure habit.

There's so much confusion around the subject, and things very often get blurred, so here's a little clarity: the idea is you start trusting yourself to make your own healthy choices and decisions about food.

Dieting is ultimately about deprivation because you end up focusing on what you shouldn't have. You can't help this; it's just part of what happens in the brain. Dieting is often driven by a set of rules where foods are either good or bad, and people become good or bad for eating them. How often do you hear someone say they were 'good' or 'bad' based on what they ate that day?

Another hallmark of dieting is its focus on weight. Dieters weigh themselves frequently and feel more and more motivated with each new pound lost. The problem is when the weight plateaus, as it always does, the motivation to follow the diet plateaus along with it. Worst of all, dieting is often followed by overeating; as we've learned throughout this book, you just can't help it.[1]

Over the years, you accumulate a lot of emotions and meanings around dieting, which is totally natural because it's such an emotional subject. When I asked my Slimpod group what dieting meant to them, they came up with lots of very sad but powerful words: misery, failure, unhappiness, fear, fixation on food, sadness, guilt, self-denial, struggle, limitations, hunger – and that was only a few!

Dieting has a lot to answer for. Of course, there are people who have success with dieting, and that's great for them. Sadly, though, they're in the minority.

## Embracing Healthy Eating Behaviours

Healthy behaviours are small changes that occur over time. Instead of following rules about good or bad foods, you learn how to balance all foods one by one. These small steps allow you to make changes that work well in your life, and this continues for as long as it takes. It hasn't got a beginning and an end like diets generally do. After dieting for years, healthy behaviours are liberating – there's no other word for it.

People who continue lifelong healthy eating are not motivated solely by weight. Instead, they appreciate how much better their lives are and, as a result, are internally motivated. Of course, weight is still a consideration, but it's far from the most important factor.

The new healthy behaviours become a preferred way to live instead of an obligation or rules to be followed. The bottom line: dieting is limiting, leaving people with few choices, while healthy behaviours expand choices, give you freedom and liberate you. As a healthy eater you love your relationship with food and think of it in an enthusiastic way – it is a friend not an enemy.

Healthy eating has substantial scientific backing. For instance, a study found that people who adopted a flexible, mindful eating approach were more successful in maintaining weight loss compared to those who followed rigid dieting rules.[2] Research has also shown that dieting can lead to long-term weight gain because of metabolic changes and psychological stress.[3]

Research in the journal *American Psychologist* indicated that diets are not only ineffective in the long run but also harmful, leading to a cycle of weight loss and regain (the dreaded yo-yo dieting).[4] Another study emphasised that restrictive diets could increase cravings and binge-eating episodes.[5] Conversely, a balanced, non-restrictive approach to eating promotes a healthier relationship with food and supports sustainable weight management.

Research reported in the *Journal of Obesity* showed that intuitive eating, which focuses on internal hunger and satiety cues rather than external diet rules, was associated with lower BMI and better psychological health.[6]

Lastly, the *New England Journal of Medicine* reported that long-term adherence to healthy eating patterns, such as the Mediterranean way, significantly reduces the risk of chronic diseases and promotes longevity.[7]

## The Mediterranean way: A path to lasting health

The Mediterranean way is not just about eating; it's a lifestyle celebrated for its health benefits. Originating from the traditional dietary patterns of countries bordering the Mediterranean Sea, it emphasises whole, natural foods and balanced eating habits. Here are the key elements:

- **Fruits and vegetables:** Abundant servings of fresh, seasonal produce.
- **Whole grains:** Including bread, pasta and cereals made from whole grains.

- **Healthy fats:** Olive oil is the primary fat source, known for its heart-healthy properties.
- **Lean proteins:** Moderate consumption of fish, poultry and legumes; limited red meat.
- **Dairy:** Moderate portions of cheese and yoghurt.
- **Nuts and seeds:** Regular consumption in small amounts.
- **Herbs and spices:** Used to flavour foods instead of salt.
- **Wine:** Consumed in moderation, typically with meals.

Why is the Mediterranean way so healthy? Because it's rich in monounsaturated fats, fibre and antioxidants, which contribute to its numerous health benefits. Studies have shown that it can reduce the risk of chronic diseases such as heart disease, diabetes and certain cancers.[8]

Additionally, its emphasis on plant-based foods and healthy fats can help to lower cholesterol levels and promote overall heart health.[9] The balanced approach to eating, combined with regular physical activity and mindful meals, supports sustainable weight management and overall well-being.

Adopting the Mediterranean way can lead to a healthier, longer life, making it a valuable choice for those seeking lasting health and vitality.

## How You Can Take Back Control

*Listen to your body*

Pay attention to your hunger and fullness cues. Eat when you're hungry and stop when you're satisfied. This simple practice can help you reconnect with your body's natural signals and prevent overeating.

*Focus on nutrient-rich foods*

Fill your plate with a variety of colourful fruits, vegetables, lean proteins and whole grains. These foods provide essential nutrients and help you feel fuller for longer. Revisit Dale Pinnock's top tips on page 71.

*Don't label foods as good or bad*

All foods can fit into a healthy diet when eaten in moderation. By avoiding strict rules and allowing yourself occasional treats, you can reduce feelings of deprivation and the likelihood of binge eating.

*Make meal planning a habit*

Planning your meals ahead of time can help you make healthier choices and avoid last-minute, less nutritious options. It also saves time and reduces stress around mealtimes.

I can hardly believe we're almost at the end of our time together. The chapters seem to have whizzed past! Hopefully I've shared so much learning with you that you're already feeling much better about yourself and are ready to lose weight and keep it off as never before. In the Conclusion – coming up next – I'll be giving you my ten pillars of wisdom. I follow them every day of my life and I hope you will, too.

## CONCLUSION

# Embrace Your Journey and Build on My Ten Pillars of Wisdom

As we reach the end of this book, I want to congratulate you on the incredible progress you've made. Whether you've already started seeing changes or you're still in the process, remember that every step you take is significant.

This journey is not about reaching a final destination, but about continuously refining your path, building habits and celebrating small wins. As you continue, I want you always to remember my ten pillars of weight-loss wisdom:

### 1. Take back control

One of the most empowering realisations is understanding that you have the power to take back control of your life. Your eating habits, relationship with food and overall well-being are within your grasp.

If your eating habits have been challenging, it's crucial to understand that this isn't a reflection of your character or willpower. Instead, it's about a system that you've developed over time, often without realising it. By acknowledging this, you can begin to change the narrative and take conscious steps towards creating healthier habits.

## 2. Use the power of small wins

Success isn't a goal to be reached or a finishing line to cross. Losing weight is a system to improve and a long-term process to refine. Celebrating small wins is an essential part of this process. Each positive change, no matter how small it may seem, contributes to your overall success.

Did you choose a healthy snack instead of something less nourishing? Did you go for a walk when you felt stressed instead of turning to comfort food? These are victories. Did you manage to drink more water today? Celebrate it. Did you choose a healthier meal? Give yourself a pat on the back. By focusing on these small wins, you build momentum and confidence.

## 3. Be consistent to build habits

Consistency is the secret sauce to sustainable success. Building new habits requires repetition and patience. Think about it: habits are formed when a new behaviour becomes automatic, like brushing your teeth or driving a car. This happens through consistent practice.

Your eating habits have developed over many years, and changing them will take time and effort. The good news is that it's entirely possible. By consistently making healthier choices, you create new neural pathways in your brain, making these choices feel more natural over time.

## 4. Well-being's a continuous process

It's important to recognise that this journey doesn't have a finish line. There's no point at which you can say: 'I've made it, and now I can stop.' Health and well-being are ongoing processes that require continuous attention and care.

By embracing this mindset, you release yourself from the pressure of achieving perfection and instead focus on progress and improvement.

## 5. Rewrite your system

Consider this: your current eating habits result from a system you might not have been fully aware of. This system includes your environment, emotional triggers and the routines you've built over time. The beauty of systems is that they can be redesigned.

By becoming aware of your triggers and making conscious choices, you can create a new, healthier system. This means setting up your environment to support your goals, finding alternative ways to cope with emotions, and establishing new routines that promote well-being.

## 6. Empower yourself with knowledge

Knowledge is power. The more you understand how your mind and body work, the better equipped you are to make positive changes. This book has provided you with so many tools and insights to help you on your journey. Continue to educate yourself, seek out information that supports your goals and apply what you learn to your daily life.

## 7. Mindset really matters

Your mindset plays a crucial role in your success. A positive mindset fuels motivation, resilience and healthier choices, making the journey enjoyable and sustainable. When you believe in yourself and maintain an optimistic outlook, setbacks become speed bumps, not roadblocks. Embrace positivity and let it guide you to a happier, healthier you.

## 8. Don't beat yourself up

Be kind to yourself. Remember, you're human not a robot, so you're allowed to have a few wobbly moments now and again. Eating a piece of chocolate doesn't mean you're a failure or that you're worthless. Self-compassion is a powerful driving force that helps keep you on the right track.

## 9. Reach out for support

Remember, you're not alone on this journey. Reach out for support when you need it. Whether it's from a friend, family member or a community of like-minded individuals, support can make a significant difference. Sharing your successes and challenges with others can provide motivation, encouragement and a sense of accountability.

## 10. It's all about you

Finally, I want to remind you that your journey towards better health and well-being is unique. It's not about comparing yourself to others or striving for an unrealistic ideal. It's about making consistent, positive changes that enhance your life. It's all about you and no one else.

By taking back control, celebrating small wins, building habits and embracing the ongoing process of improvement, you are on the path to a healthier, happier you.

Success is not a destination; it's a journey. And you are well on your way. Keep moving forward, stay positive and remember that every step you take is a step towards a better, more empowered version of yourself.

# Bibliography

*Altered Traits*, Daniel Goleman and Richard J. Davidson (Avery Publishing Group, Inc., 2018)

*Atomic Habits*, James Clear (Random House Business, 2018)

*Blink*, Malcolm Gladwell (Penguin, 2006)

*Brain Rules*, John Medina (Pear Press, 2014)

*Change Your Brain, Change Your Body*, Dr Daniel G. Amen (Piatkus, 2012)

*Deep Work*, Cal Newport (Piatkus, 2016)

*Drive*, Daniel H. Pink (Canongate Books, 2018)

*Emotional Intelligence*, Daniel Goleman (Bloomsbury Publishing, 2020)

*Flourish*, Martin Seligman (Nicholas Brealey Publishing, 2011)

*Food Rules*, Michael Pollan (Penguin, 2010)

*Good Calories, Bad Calories*, Gary Taubes (Vintage, 2008)

*Grit*, Angela Duckworth (Vermilion, 2017)

*How Emotions Are Made*, Lisa Feldman Barrett (Pan, 2018)

*How the Mind Works*, Steven Pinker (Penguin, 2015)

*Incognito*, David Eagleman (Canongate Canons, 2016)

*Influence*, Robert B. Cialdini (Harper Business, 2021)

*Intuitive Eating*, Evelyn Tribole and Elyse Resch (Essentials, 2020)

*Mindless Eating*, Brian Wansink (Bantam, 2007)

*Mindset*, Carol S. Dweck (Random House Publishing Group, 2007)

*Nudge*, Richard H. Thaler and Cass R. Sunstein (Penguin, 2022)

*Predictably Irrational*, Dan Ariely (Harper, 2009)

*Presence*, Amy Cuddy (Orion Spring, 2023)

*Rewire Your Brain*, John B. Arden (Wiley, 2010)

*Self-Compassion*, Kristin Neff (Yellow Kite, 2011)

*Self-Efficacy*, Albert Bandura (Worth Publishers, 1997)
*Self-Regulated Learning and Academic Achievement*, Barry J.
   Zimmerman and Dale Schunk (Routledge, 2001)
*Spark*, Dr John J. Ratey and Eric Hagerman (Quercus, 2010)
*Switch*, Chip and Dan Heath (Random House Business, 2011)
*The Biology of Belief*, Bruce H. Lipton (Hay House UK, 2015)
*The Brain That Changes Itself*, Norman Doidge (Penguin, 2008)
*The Compass of Pleasure*, David J. Linden (Viking, 2011)
*The Definitive Guide to the Perimenopause and Menopause*, Dr Louise
   Newson (Yellow Kite, 2024)
*The Diet Myth*, Tim Spector (Weidenfeld & Nicolson, 2016)
*The End of Overeating*, David A. Kessler (Penguin, 2010)
*The Genie in Your Genes*, Dawson Church (Energy Psychology Press,
   2009)
*The Gifts of Imperfection*, Brené Brown (Hazelden Publishing &
   Educational Services, 2022)
*The Happiness Advantage*, Shawn Achor (Virgin Books, 2011)
*The Hungry Brain*, Stephan J. Guyenet (Vermilion, 2017)
*The Mind–Gut Connection*, Emeran Mayer (Harper, 2018)
*The Neuroscience of Change*, Kelly McGonigal [audio] (Sounds True)
*The Power of Habit*, Charles Duhigg (Random House Books, 2013)
*The Power of Your Subconscious Mind*, Dr Joseph Murphy (Simon &
   Schuster UK, 2019)
*The Psychobiotic Revolution*, Scott C. Anderson with John F. Cryan
   and Ted Dinan (National Geographic, 2019)
*The Secret Life of the Mind*, Mariano Sigman (William Collins, 2018)
*The Talent Code*, Daniel Coyle (Random House Business, 2020)
*The Upside of Stress*, Kelly McGonigal (Vermilion, 2015)
*The Upward Spiral*, Alex Korb (New Harbinger, 2015)
*The Willpower Instinct*, Kelly McGonigal (Avery Publishing Group,
   Inc., 2013)
*Thinking, Fast and Slow*, Daniel Kahneman (Penguin, 2012)
*Thinking in Bets*, Annie Duke (Portfolio, 2018)
*Willpower*, Roy F. Baumeister and John Tierney (Penguin, 2012)
*Your Brain at Work*, Dr David Rock (Harper Business, 2020)

# Acknowledgements

With huge gratitude to the 3,879 Slimpodders who took part in my groundbreaking survey on the psychological effects of dieting. They inspired me to write this book.

And special thanks to all those people who have allowed me to share their deeply personal stories on these pages: Dr Victoria Baxter, Ava Brodie, Rachael Buckett, John Burns, Ellie Cadwallader White, Vivienne Chapman, Charlotte Donovan, Jane Foster, Lyn Fox, Ronnie Gregory, Lynn Haddrell, Jane Harman, Poppy Hinton, Heather Manning, Michelle Marshall, Darin McCloud, Colette Molloy, Lorraine Murphy, Biddy O'Sullivan, Clare Rayner, Caroline R, Tanya Wakeford and June Ward. Without their courage and openness, this book would not have been possible.

Thanks you to my publisher Carolyn Thorne, without whom this book wouldn't have been written. She believed the world needed it and she empowered me every step of the way. Thanks also to the rest of the Yellow Kite team, Zoe Maple, assistant editor and Julia Kellaway for the copyediting.

Finally, thanks to my husband Chris, for his huge support.

# Endnotes

## Introduction

1. Baker, C. 'Obesity statistics' House of Commons Library (12 Jan. 2023). Retrieved from https://researchbriefings.files.parliament. uk/documents/SN03336/SN03336.pdf.
2. World Health Organization 'Obesity and overweight: Factsheet' (1 Mar. 2024). Retrieved from https://www.who.int/news-room/fact-sheets/detail/obesity-and-overweight.
3. Okunogbe, A. et al. 'Economic impacts of overweight and obesity: Current and future estimates for 161 countries' *BMJ Global Health* 7.9 (2022): e009773.
4. Stunkard, A. J. & McLaren-Hume, M. 'The results of treatment for obesity' *Pennsylvania School of Medicine* (1959).
5. Memon, S. et al. 'Obesity management: A review' California Institute of Behavioral Neurosciences & Psychology, *National Library of Medicine* (2020).
6. Freedhoff, Y. *The Diet Fix: Why everything you've been taught about dieting is wrong and the 10-day plan to fix it* (Harmony Books, 2014).
7. Mann, T. et al. 'Medicare's search for effective obesity treatments: Diets are not the answer' *American Psychologist* 62.3 (2007): 220–33.

## Chapter 1: Why 85 Per Cent of People Self-Sabotage

1. Lowe, M. R. et al. 'Dieting and restrained eating as prospective predictors of weight gain' *Frontiers in Psychology* 4 (2013): 577.
2. Teixeira, P. J. et al. 'Why we eat what we eat: The role of autonomous motivation in eating behaviour regulation' *International Journal of Behavioural Nutrition and Physical Activity* 7 (2010): 78.

3. Linde, J. A. et al. 'Weight loss goals and treatment outcomes among overweight men and women enrolled in a weight loss trial' *International Journal of Obesity* 29 (2005): 1002–5.
4. Neal, D. T. et al. 'Habitual behaviour and the effects of stress' *Journal of Personality and Social Psychology* 101.4 (2011): 925–36.

## Chapter 2: Don't Let the Scales Dictate Your Mood
1. Kahneman, D. & Tversky, A. 'The psychology of prediction' *Psychological Review* 80.4 (1973): 237–51.
2. Thompson, J. K. & Pasman, L. 'Psychological consequences of frequent weighing' *Journal of Psychosomatic Research* 53.5 (2002): 993–5.

## Chapter 3: Ending an Obsession With Food
1. Parent, M. B. & Darling, J. N. 'Remembering to eat: Hippocampal regulation of meal onset' *American Journal of Physiology* 306.4 (2014): R301–10.
2. Carr, K. D. 'Reward-related neuroadaptations induced by food restriction: Pathogenic potential of a survival mechanism' *Obesity Prevention* (2010): 65–84.
3. Polivy, J. 'Psychological consequences of food restriction' *Journal of the Academy of Nutrition and Dietetics* 96.6 (1996): 589–95.
4. Erskine, J. A. et al. 'The forbidden fruit effect: Cognitive control of eating and its motivational consequences' *Appetite* 54.3 (2010): 481–6.
5. Cummings, D. E. & Overduin, J. 'Ghrelin and leptin: Physiology and pathophysiology' *Journal of Clinical Endocrinology & Metabolism* 92.9 (2007): 3554–61.
6. Kristeller, J. L, & Wolever, R. Q. 'Mindfulness-based eating awareness training for treating binge eating disorder: The conceptual foundation' *Eating Disorders* 19.1 (2011): 49–61.

## Chapter 4: Cravings: Dieting's Hidden Side Effect
1. Polivy, J. & Herman, C. P. 'Dieting and binge eating: A causal analysis' *American Psychologist* 40.2 (1985): 193–201.
2. Volkow, N. D. et al. 'Obesity: Psychological and behavioural aspects' *Journal of Clinical Investigation* 110.4 (2002): 555–64.

3. Wansink, B. & Sobal, J. 'Mindless eating: The 200 daily food decisions we overlook' *Environment and Behavior* 39.1 (2007): 106–23.
4. Baumeister, R. F. et al. 'Self-regulation and eating behaviour' *Psychological Inquiry* 5.3 (1994): 19—205.
5. Tylka, T. L. et al. 'Intuitive eating scale: Development and validation' *Journal of Counselling Psychology* 53.2 (2006): 226–40.
6. Neff, K. D. 'Self-compassion: An alternative conceptualisation of a healthy attitude toward oneself' *Self and Identity* 2.2 (2003): 85–101.
7. Story, M. et al. 'Creating healthy food and eating environments: Policy and environmental approaches' *Annual Review of Public Health* 29 (2008): 253–72.

## Chapter 5: Overcoming Self-Limiting Beliefs

1. Conner, T. S. & Barrett, L. F. 'Implicit self-attitudes predict spontaneous affect in daily life' *Emotion* 5.4 (2005): 476–88.
2. Rudman, L. A. 'Sources of implicit attitudes' *Current Directions in Psychological Science* 13.2 (2004): 79–82.
3. Olson, M. A. & Fazio, R. H. 'Implicit acquisition and manifestation of classically conditioned attitude' *Social Cognition* 20.2 (2002): 89–104.
4. Pearce, A. 'Reframing self-limiting beliefs' *The Open University* (19 Aug. 2021). Retrieved from https://www.open.edu/openlearn/course/view.php?id=15395.

## Chapter 6: The Hidden Impact of Dieting on Self-Esteem

1. Polivy, J. & Herman, C. P. 'Dieting and binge eating: A causal analysis' *American Psychologist* 40.2 (1985): 193–201.
2. Heatherton, T. F. et al. 'Chronic dieting and self-esteem' *Journal of Personality and Social Psychology* 60.1 (1991): 56–70.
3. Festinger, L. 'A theory of social comparison processes' *Human Relations* 7.2 (1954): 117–40.
4. Groesz, L. M. et al. 'The effect of experimental presentation of thin media images on body satisfaction: A meta-analytic review' *International Journal of Eating Disorders* 31.1 (2002): 1–16.
5. Festinger, L. *A Theory of Cognitive Dissonance* (Stanford University Press, 1957).
6. Neff, K. D. 'Self-compassion: An alternative conceptualisation of a healthy attitude toward oneself' *Self and Identity* 2.2 (2003): 85–101.

## Chapter 7: Breaking Through Fear: Your Path to Success

1. Jones, D. 'Fear of weight regain: A study' *Obesity Research Journal* 25.1 (2017): 55–62.
2. Smith, E. M. 'Psychological impact of weight loss' *Journal of Health Psychology* 23.4 (2018): 489–98.
3. Lee, S. 'Anticipatory anxiety and weight management' *Weight Psychology Review* 9.2 (2019): 133–45.
4. Brown, K. J. 'Behavioural responses to weight loss fear' *Clinical Psychology Review* 31.2 (2020): 120–34.

## Chapter 8: Factory Food Is Making the World Fatter

1. Cordova, R. et al. 'Consumption of ultra-processed foods associated with weight gain and obesity in adults' *Clinical Nutrition* 40.9 (2021): 5079–88.
2. NHS England. 'Health Survey for England, 2021, part 1' (15 Dec. 2022). Retrieved from https://digital.nhs.uk/data-and-information/publications/statistical/health-survey-for-england/2021.
3. https://www.cdc.gov/obesity/adult-obesity-facts/index.html.
4. La Berge, A. F. 'How the ideology of low fat conquered America' *Journal of the History of Medicine and Allied Sciences* 63.2 (2008): 139–77.
5. Lenoir, M. et al. 'Intense sweetness surpasses cocaine reward' *PloS One* 2.8 (2007): e698.
6. Nguyen, T. et al. 'A systematic comparison of sugar content in low-fat vs regular versions of food' *Nutrition & Diabetes* 6 (2016): e193.
7. Teff, K. L. et al. 'Dietary fructose reduces circulating insulin and leptin, attenuates postprandial suppression of ghrelin, and increases triglycerides in women' *The Journal of Clinical Endocrinology & Metabolism* 89.6 (2004): 2963–72.
8. Johnson, R. J. 'The fructose survival hypothesis for obesity' *Philosophical Transactions of the Royal Society B: Biological Sciences* 378.1874 (2023): 20220230.
9. DeChristopher, L. R. et al. 'Intake of high fructose corn syrup sweetened soft drinks' *BMC Nutrition* 3.1 (2017): 12–23.
10. Prada, M. et al. 'Perceived associations between excessive sugar intake and health conditions' *Nutrients* 14.3 (2022): 640.
11. Donnelly, L. & Taylor, R. 'Major food companies "acting like Big Tobacco" by selling addictive and harmful products.' *Daily Telegraph* (9 Dec. 2023).

## Chapter 9: The Hidden Hurdle of Addictions

1. Avena, N. M. et al. 'Evidence for sugar addiction: Behavioral and neurochemical effects of intermittent, excessive sugar intake' *Neuroscience & Biobehavioral Reviews* 32.1 (2008): 20–39.
2. Volkow, N. D. et al. 'Reward, dopamine, and the control of food intake: Implications for obesity' *Trends in Cognitive Science* 15.1 (2011): 37–46.
3. Volkow, N. D. et al. 'The addictive dimensionality of obesity' *Nature Neuroscience* 10.5 (2007): 535–6.
4. Goldstein, R. Z. & Volkow, N. D. 'Drug addiction and its underlying neurobiological basis: Neuroimaging evidence for the involvement of the frontal cortex' *American Journal of Psychiatry* 159.10 (2002): 1642–52.
5. Carroll, K. M. & Onken, L. S. 'Behavioral therapies for drug abuse' *American Journal of Psychiatry* 162.8 (2005): 1452–60.
6. Brown, R. A. et al. 'Aerobic exercise for alcohol recovery: Rationale, program description, and preliminary findings' *Behaviour Modification* 36.1 (2012): 37–55.


## Chapter 10: Why Dieting Makes Weight Loss Harder

1. Dulloo, A. G. & Montani, J. P. 'Pathways from dieting to weight regain, to obesity and to the metabolic syndrome: An overview' *Obesity Reviews* 16 (2015): 1–6.
2. Sumithran, P. et al. 'Long-term persistence of hormonal adaptations to weight loss' *New England Journal of Medicine* 365.17 (2011): 1597–1604.
3. Kaisinger, J. L. et al. 'New genes linked to obesity in large study' *Cell Genomics* 1.2 (2023): 102–13.
4. Fothergill, E. et al. 'Persistent metabolic adaptation 6 years after The Biggest Loser competition' *Obesity (Silver Spring)* 24.8 (2016): 1612–19.


## Chapter 11: Navigating the Menopause Minefield

1. Collins, P. et al. 'Estrogen and hormone replacement therapy: Current controversies' *Women's Health* 8.3 (2012): 325–34.
2. Cummings, D. E. & Overduin, J. 'Ghrelin and metabolic control: Weight loss, obesity, and hormone replacement therapy' *Gastroenterology* 132.6 (2007): 2088–100.
3. Finer, N. & Bloom, S. R. 'Hormonal regulation of appetite and weight loss' *International Journal of Obesity* 35 (2011): 12–20.

4. Adam, T. C. & Epel, E. S. 'Stress, eating, and the reward system' *Physiology & Behavior* 91.4 (2007): 449–58.
5. Van Dijk, G. & Smit, J. 'Neuroendocrinology of the reward system and the regulation of food intake' *Annals of the New York Academy of Sciences* 1212 (2011): 131–48.
6. Collins, P. et al. 'Estrogen and hormone replacement therapy: Current controversies' *Women's Health* 8.3 (2012): 325–34.
7. Newson, L. *Definitive Guide to the Perimenopause and Menopause* (Yellow Kite, 2024).
8. Cummings, D. E. & Overduin, J. 'Ghrelin and metabolic control: Weight loss, obesity, and hormone replacement therapy' *Gastroenterology* 132.6 (2007): 2088–100.
9. Collins, P. et al. 'Estrogen and hormone replacement therapy: Current controversies' *Women's Health* 8.3 (2012): 325–34.
10. Tresserra-Rimbau, A, & Hurtado-Barroso, S. 'Effects of dietary phytoestrogens on hormones throughout a human lifespan: A review' *Nutrients* 12.8 (2020): 2456.

## Chapter 12: How Stress Increases Tummy Fat

1. Kirschbaum, C. et al. 'The Trier social stress test – A tool for investigating psychobiological stress responses in a laboratory setting' *Neuropsychobiology* 28.1-2 (1993): 76–81.
2. Epel, E. S. et al. 'Stress and body shape: Stress-induced cortisol secretion is consistently greater among women with central fat' *Psychosomatic Medicine* 62.5 (2000): 623–32.
3. Kiecolt-Glaser, J. K. et al. 'Stress, food, and inflammation: Psychoneuroimmunology and nutrition at the cutting edge' *Psychosomatic Medicine* 72.4 (2010): 365–9.
4. McEwen, B. S. 'Protective and damaging effects of stress mediators.' *New England Journal of Medicine* 338.3 (1998): 171–9.
5. Dallman, M. F. et al. 'Chronic stress and comfort foods: Self-medication and abdominal obesity' *Brain, Behavior, and Immunity* 19.4 (2005): 275–80.
6. Gu, J. et al. 'How do mindfulness-based cognitive therapy and mindfulness-based stress reduction improve mental health and wellbeing? A systematic review and meta-analysis of mediation studies' *Clinical Psychology Review* 37 (2015): 1–12.
7. Neumann J et al, "The impact of physical fitness on resilience to modern life stress and the mediating role of general self-efficacy," (2021) European Archives of Psychiatry and Clinical Neuroscience

271(3), 449–457. https://url.de.m.mimecastprotect.com/s/32x2COg WXASpxL9WIvhPIGU5Cc?domain=doi.org.

8. Spiegel, K. et al. 'Impact of sleep debt on metabolic and endocrine function.' The Lancet 354.9188 (1999): 1435–9.

## Chapter 13: Poor Sleep Sabotages Weight Loss

1. Chaput, J. P. & Tremblay, A. 'Sleeping habits predict the magnitude of fat loss in adults exposed to moderate caloric restriction' Obesity Facts 5.1 (2012): 56–65.
2. Revonsuo, A. 'Consciousness, dreams, and virtual realities' Philosophical Psychology 8.1 (1995): 35–58.
3. Broussard, J. 'Impact of sleep deprivation on insulin sensitivity' Journal of Clinical Endocrinology & Metabolism 103.1 (2018): 1–8.
4. Greer, S. M. et al. 'The impact of sleep deprivation on food desire in the human brain' Nature Communications 4 (2013): 1–7.
5. Smith, E. M. 'Emotional eating: Understanding the triggers and solutions' Journal of Health Psychology 24.7 (2019): 865–79.
6. Brown, K. J. 'The role of stress and eating behaviours in weight gain' Clinical Nutrition 35.4 (2020): 1049–61.
7. Ibid.

## Chapter 14: Drive a Wedge Into Emotional Eating

1. Canetti, L. et al. 'Food and emotion' Behavioural Processes 60.2 (2002): 157–64.
2. Masheb, R. M. & Grilo, C. M. 'Emotional overeating and its associations with eating disorder psychopathology among overweight patients with binge eating disorder' International Journal of Eating Disorders 39 (2006): 141–6.
3. Thompson, R. 'Stress and child development' The Future of Children 24.1 (2014): 41–59.
4. Ljubičić, M. et al. 'Emotions and food consumption: emotional eating behavior in a European population.' Foods 12.4 (2023): 872.
5. Bohon, C. et al. 'Low self-esteem as a risk factor for emotional eating in adolescents' International Journal of Eating Disorders 42.2 (2009): 142–50.
6. Macht, M. 'How emotions affect eating: A five-way model' Appetite 50.1 (2008): 1–11.
7. Gibson, E. L. 'Emotional influences on food choice: Sensory,

physiological and psychological pathways' *Physiology & Behavior,* 89.1 (2006): 53–61.

8. Appelhans, B. M. 'Neurobehavioral inhibition of reward-driven feeding: Implications for dieting and obesity.' *Obesity* 17.4 (2009): 640–7.

9. Adam, T. C. & Epel, E. S. 'Stress, eating and the reward system' *Physiology & Behavior,* 91.4 (2007): 449–58.

10. Volkow, N. D. et al. 'Reward, dopamine, and the control of food intake: Implications for obesity' *Trends in Cognitive Sciences,* 15.1 (2011): 37–46.

11. Kiecolt-Glaser, J. K. et al. 'Chronic stress and age-related increases in the proinflammatory cytokine IL-6' *Proceedings of the National Academy of Sciences,* 100.15 (2003): 9090–5.

12. Felitti, V. J. et al. 'Relationship of childhood abuse and household dysfunction to many of the leading causes of death in adults: The adverse childhood experiences (ACE) study' *American Journal of Preventive Medicine* 14.4 (1998): 245–58.

## Chapter 15: Escape From a Mental Groove

1. Melzer, T. M. et al. 'Exploring the role of neuroplasticity in development, aging, and neurodegeneration' *Brain Sciences* 13.1 (2023): 35–44.

2. Volkow, N. D. et al. 'Food and drug rewards: Overlapping circuits in human obesity and addiction' *Current Topics in Behavioral Neurosciences* 11 (2011): 1–13.

3. Larimer, M. E. et al. 'Relapse prevention: An overview of Marlatt's cognitive-behavioral model' *Alcohol Research & Health* 23.2 (1988): 131–41.

4. Neff, K. 'Self-compassion: An alternative conceptualization of a healthy attitude toward oneself' *Self and Identity* 2.2 (2003): 85–101.

## Chapter 16: Challenge Your Distorted Thoughts About Food

1. Beck, A. T. *Cognitive Therapy and the Emotional Disorders* (International Universities Press, 1976).

2. Polivy, J. and Herman, C. P. 'Dieting and binge eating: A causal analysis' *American Psychologist* 40.2 (1985): 193–201.

3. Beck, A. T. & Emery, G. *Anxiety Disorders and Phobias: A cognitive perspective* (Basic Books, 1985).

4. Sullivan, M. J. L. et al. 'Theoretical perspectives on the relation between catastrophizing and pain' *The Clinical Journal of Pain* 17.1 (2001): 52–64.
5. Gilbert, P. *Overcoming Depression: A self-help guide using cognitive behavioral techniques* (Constable & Robinson, 2009).
6. Morrison, A. S. & Heimberg, R. G. 'Social anxiety and eating disorder behaviors: The role of negative social evaluation fears' *Eating Behaviors*, 9.4 (2008): 407–12.
7. Svaldi, J. et al. 'The effects of emotions on eating behavior: A comparison of emotional reasoning and emotional eating' *Appetite*, 58.3 (2012): 785–90.
8. Rosenfield, M. & Smillie, L. D. 'Becoming aware: Cognitive awareness and the reduction of distorted thinking in emotional regulation' *Cognitive Therapy and Research*, 38.4 (2014): 418–25.
9. Beck, A. T. & Dozois, D. J. A. 'Cognitive therapy: Current status and future directions' *Annual Review of Medicine*, 62 (2011): 397–409.
10. Neff, K. D. *Self-compassion: The proven power of being kind to yourself* (William Morrow, 2011).

## Chapter 17: Tame Your Inner Critic, Transform Your Inner Voice

1. Baumeister, R. F. et al. 'Bad is stronger than good' *Review of General Psychology* 5.4 (2001): 323–70.
2. Sheline, Y. I. et al. 'The default mode network and self-referential processes in depression' *Proceedings of the National Academy of Sciences* 106.6 (2009): 1942–7.
3. Gilbert, P. & Procter, S. 'Compassionate mind training for people with high shame and self-criticism' *Clinical Psychology & Psychotherapy* 13.6 (2006): 353–79.

## Chapter 18: Rewire Your Habits: The Secret to Lasting Change

1. Orbell, S. & Verplanken, B. 'The automatic component of habit in health behaviour: Habit as cue-contingent automaticity' *American Health Psychology* 29.4 (2010): 374–83.
2. Bruner, J. S. 'Repetition is the first principle of all learning' *University of Virginia, ResearchGate* (2001): 1–16.
3. Orbell, S. & Verplanken, B. 'The automatic component of habit in

health behaviour: Habit as cue-contingent automaticity' *Health Psychology* 29.4 (2010): 374–83.

4. Gardner, B. et al. 'Developing habit-based health behaviour change interventions' *Psychology & Health* 36.5 (2021): 591–608.

5. Smith, E. M. et al. 'Reversible online control of habitual behaviour' *Proceedings of the National Academy of Sciences* 109.14 (2012): 592–9.

6. Aldao, A. et al. 'Emotion-regulation strategies across psychopathology: A meta-analytic review' *Clinical Psychology Review* 30.2 (2010): 217–37.

7. Draganski, B. et al. 'Temporal and spatial dynamics of brain structure changes during extensive learning' *Journal of Neuroscience* 26.23 (2006): 6314–17.

8. Fogg, B. J. 'A behavior model for persuasive design' In: *Proceedings of the 4th International Conference on Persuasive Technology* (ACM, 2009): 1–7.

9. Ibid.

10. Ibid.

11. Taylor, S. E. & Pham, L. B. 'Mental simulation, motivation, and action' *Journal of Personality and Social Psychology* 69.5 (1996): 841–52.

## Chapter 19: Unlock the Power of Anchors

1. Pavlov, I. P. *Conditioned Reflexes: An investigation of the physiological activity of the cerebral cortex* (Oxford University Press, 1927).

2. Wood, W. & Neal, D. T. 'A new look at habits and the habit-goal interface' *Psychological Review* 114.4 (2007): 843–63.

3. Doidge, N. *The Brain That Changes Itself: Stories of personal triumph from the frontiers of brain science* (Penguin, 2007).

4. Heatherton, T. F. & Baumeister, R. F. 'Binge eating as escape from self-awareness' *Psychological Bulletin* 110.1 (1991): 86–108.

## Chapter 20: Overcome Guilt – The Silent Saboteur

1. Press Association. 'Women own up to guilt over eating habits' *Guardian* (20 Jan. 2013).

2. Taylor, R. D. 'The role of guilt in binge eating' *Appetite* 144 (2020): 104486.

3. Brown, K. J. 'Food guilt and mental health in dieting adults' *Psychology of Eating Behaviours* 33.1 (2019): 29–38.

4. Polivy, J. & Herman, C. P. 'Dieting and binging: A causal analysis' *American Psychologist* 40.2 (1985): 193–201.

5. Keys, A. et al. *The Biology of Human Starvation* (University of Minnesota Press, 1950).
6. Wolpe, J. *Psychotherapy by Reciprocal Inhibition* (Stanford University Press, 1958).
7. Tylka, T. L. 'Development and psychometric evaluation of a measure of intuitive eating' *Journal of Counseling Psychology* 53.2 (2006): 226–40.
8. Kristeller, J. L. & Wolever, R. Q. 'Mindfulness-based eating awareness training for treating binge eating disorder: The conceptual foundation' *Eating Disorders* 19.1 (2011): 49–61.
9. Neff, K. 'Self-compassion: An alternative conceptualization of a healthy attitude toward oneself' *Self and Identity* 2.2 (2003): 85–101.
10. Adams, C. E. & Leary, M. R. 'Promoting self-compassionate attitudes toward eating among restrictive and guilty eaters' *Journal of Social and Clinical Psychology* 26.10 (2007): 1120–44.

## Chapter 21: Stop Your Mind Fighting Against You

1. Cooper, J. *Cognitive Dissonance: Fifty years of a classic theory* (Sage Publications, 2007).
2. Kavanagh, D. J. et al. 'Imaginary relish and exquisite torture: The elaborated intrusion theory of desire' *Psychological Review* 112.2 (2005): 446–7.

## Chapter 22: Avoid the Willpower Trap

1. Wansink, B. & Sobal, J. 'Mindless eating: The 200 food decisions we overlook' *Environment and Behavior* 39.1 (2007): 106–23.
2. Baumeister, R. F. et al. 'Self-regulation, ego depletion, and inhibition' *Neuropsychologia* 65 (2014): 313–19.
3. Saunders, B. et al. 'The impact of stress on brain functions related to self-control' *Journal of Neuroscience* 38.5 (2018): 1415–25.
4. Festinger, L. *A Theory of Cognitive Dissonance* (Stanford University Press, 1957).
5. Polivy, J. et al. 'The effect of deprivation on food cravings and eating behavior in restrained and unrestrained eaters' *International Journal of Eating Disorders* 38.3 (2005): 301–9.
6. Loewenstein, G. 'Insights on how immediate desires overpower long-term goals' *Journal of Consumer Research* 17.1 (1991): 78–91.
7. McClure, S. M, et al. 'Separate neural systems value immediate and delayed monetary rewards' *Science* 306.5695 (2004): 503–7.

8. Tice, D. M. et al. 'Emotional distress regulation takes precedence over impulse control: If you feel bad, do it!' *Journal of Personality & Social Psychology*, 80.1 (2001): 53–67.
9. Baumeister, R. F. et al. 'Ego depletion: Is the active self a limited resource?' *Journal of Personality and Social Psychology* 74.5 (1998): 1252–65.

## Chapter 23: Sidestep the Influence of Marketing Tricks

1. Chandon, P. et al, 'Does in-store marketing work? Effects of the number and position of shelf facings on brand attention and evaluation at the point of purchase' *Journal of Marketing*, (2009): 73(6), 1–17.
2. Bargh, J. A. et al. 'Automaticity of social behavior: Direct effects of trait construct and stereotype activation on action' *Journal of Personality and Social Psychology* 71.2 (1996): 230–44.
3. Ibid.
4. Bargh, J. A. & Chartrand, T. L., 'The unbearable automaticity of being' *American Psychologist* 54.7 (1999): 462–79.
5. Janiszewski, C. 'Preattentive mere exposure effects' *Journal of Consumer Research*, 20.3 (2003): 376–92.
6. Harris, J. L. et al. 'Priming effects of television food advertising on eating behavior' *Health Psychology* 28.4 (2009): 404–13.
7. Rawn, C. D. & Vohs, K. D. 'People use their friends to manage their goals' *Journal of Personality and Social Psychology* 100.6 (2011): 1044–56.
8. Elliot, A. J. & Maier, M. A. 'Color and psychological functioning: The effect of red on performance attainment' *Journal of Experimental Psychology* 136.1 (2007): 154–68.
9. Higgins, E. T. & King, G. 'Accessibility of social constructs: Information-processing consequences of individual and contextual variability' *Personality, Cognition, and Social Interaction* 3 (1981), 69–121.
10. Goldstein, N. J. et al. 'A room with a viewpoint: Using social norms to motivate environmental conservation in hotels' *Journal of Consumer Research* 35.3 (2008): 472–82.
11. Strahan, E. et al., 'Subliminal priming and persuasion: Striking while the iron is hot' *Journal of Experimental Social Psychology* 38 (2002): 556–68.

## Chapter 24: Launch Your Brain's Goal-Seeking Missile

1. Posner, M. I. 'Attention: The mechanisms of consciousness' *Proceedings of the National Academy of Sciences* 108.1 (2011): 1910–12.
2. Lane, R. D. & Nadel, L. *The Cognitive Neuroscience of Emotion* (Oxford University Press, 2000).
3. Matthews, G. 'Writing goals makes them more effective. Dominican University of California (2007): 1–18.
4. Kyllo, L. B. & Landers, D. M. 'Goal setting in sport and exercise: A research synthesis to resolve the controversy' *Journal of Sport and Exercise Psychology* 17.2 (1995): 117–37.

## Chapter 25: Identify the 'Big Why' of Weight Loss

1. Cole, S, et al. 'Motivation and physiology influence distance perception' *Journal of Experimental Psychology* 142.1 (2013): 18–22.
2. Berkman, E. T. 'The neuroscience of goals and behavior change' *Consulting Psychology Journal* 70.1 (2018): 28–44.
3. Pascual-Leone, A. et al. 'Modulation of muscle responses evoked by transcranial magnetic stimulation during the acquisition of new fine motor skills' *Journal of Neurophysiology* 74.3 (1995): 1037–45.
4. Berkman, E. T. 'The neuroscience of goals and behavior change' *Consulting Psychology Journal: Practice and Research* 70.1 (2018): 28–44.
5. Laguna, M. et al. 'Personal goal realisation in entrepreneurs: A multilevel analysis of the role of affect and positive orientation' *Applied Psychology* 65.3 (2016): 599–620.
6. Berkman, E. T. 'The neuroscience of goals and behavior change' *Consulting Psychology Journal: Practice and Research* 70.1 (2018): 28–44.

## Chapter 26: Picture Your Success:
## The Role of Visualisation

1. Horowitz, M. J. 'Visualisation and goal achievement: The role of mental imagery in success' *Journal of Applied Psychology* 95.2 (2010): 195–208.
2. Guillot, A. & Collet, C. 'Construction of the motor imagery integrative model in sport: A review and theoretical investigation of motor imagery use' *International Review of Sport and Exercise Psychology* 1.1 (2008): 31–44.

3. Taylor, S. E. & Pham, L. B. 'The effect of mental imagery on motivation and performance' *Journal of Consulting and Clinical Psychology* 65.2 (1997): 248-257.
4. Kosslyn, S. M. *Image and Brain: The resolution of the imagery debate* (MIT Press, 1994).
5. Martin, K. A. et al. 'Imagery use in sport: A literature review and applied model' *The Sport Psychologist* 13.3 (1999): 245–268.
6. Feltz, D. L. & Landers, D. M., 'The effects of mental practice on motor skill learning and performance: A meta-analysis' *Journal of Sport Psychology* 5.1 (1983): 25–57.
7. Guillot, A. & Collet, C. 'Construction of the motor imagery integrative model in sport: A review and theoretical investigation of motor imagery use' *International Review of Sport and Exercise Psychology*, 1.1 (2008): 31–44.

## Chapter 27: Become the Internal Master of Your Life

1. Rotter, J. B. 'Generalized expectancies for internal versus external control of reinforcement' *Psychological Monographs: General and Applied* 80.1 (1966): 1–28.
2. Lefcourt, H. M. *Locus of Control: Current trends in theory and research* (Lawrence Erlbaum Associates, 1976).
3. Spector, P. E. 'Development of the work locus of control scale' *Journal of Occupational Psychology* 61.4 (1988): 335–40.
4. Gale, C. R. et al. 'Locus of control at age 10 years and health outcomes and behaviours at age 30 years: The 1970 British cohort study' *Psychosomatic Medicine* 70.4 (2008): 397–403.
5. Ng, K. Y., Ang, S. & Chan, K. Y. 'Personality and leader effectiveness: A moderated mediation model of leadership self-efficacy, job demands, and job autonomy' *Journal of Applied Psychology* 93.4 (2008): 733–43.

## Chapter 28: Be a 'Can Do' Person: The Power of Belief

1. Bandura, A. *Self-efficacy: The exercise of control* (W.H. Freeman and Company, 1997).
2. Ibid.
3. Zimmerman, B. J. & Schunk, D. H. *Self-regulated Learning and Performance* (Routledge, 2012).
4. Pajares, F. 'Self-efficacy beliefs in academic settings' *Review of Educational Research* 66.4 (1996): 543–78.

5. Schwarzer, R. 'Self-efficacy in the adoption and maintenance of health behaviors' In *Self-efficacy: Though control of action* 43.2 (1992): 231–47.
6. Baumeister, R. F. & Heatherton, T. F. 'Self-regulation failure: An overview' *Psychological Inquiry* 7.1 (1996): 1–15.
7. Dweck, C. S. *Mindset: The new psychology of success* (Random House Publishing Group, 2006).
8. Bandura, A. 'Self-efficacy: Toward a unifying theory of behavioral change' *Psychological Review* 84.2 (1977): 191–215.
9. Deci, E. L. & Ryan, R. M. 'Self-determination theory: An approach to human motivation and personality' *American Psychologist* 55 (2001): 68–78.
10. Bennett, J. et al. 'Perceptions of emotional eating behavior: A qualitative study of college students' *Journal of Nutrition Education and Behavior* 45.6 (2013): 554–60.
11. Deci, E. L., & Ryan, R. M. *Intrinsic Motivation and Self-Determination in Human Behavior* (Springer Science & Business Media, 2013).
12. Bandura, A. *Self-Efficacy: The exercise of control* (W.H. Freeman, 1997).
13. Ibid.
14. Weinberg, R. S. & Gould, D. 'Imagery in sport and exercise: Development, measurement, and applications' *International Journal of Sport and Exercise Psychology* (2010).
15. Weinberg, R. S. et al. 'Mental preparation strategies, cognitions, and strength performance' *Journal of Sport Psychology* 2 (1980): 329–39.
16. Matthews, G. 'Writing goals makes them more effective' Dominican University of California (2007): 1–18.

## Chapter 29: Harness the Power of a Growth Mindset

1. Dweck, C. S. *Mindset: The new psychology of success* (Random House Publishing Group, 2006).
2. Howell, A. J. & Shepperd, J. A. 'Reducing the harms of self-set goals: The benefits of implementation intentions' *Journal of Applied Psychology* 97.3 (2012): 754–62.
3. Aronson, J. et al. 'Reducing the effects of stereotype threat on African American college students by shaping theories of intelligence' *Journal of Experimental Social Psychology* 38.2 (2002): 113–25.
4. Paunesku, D. et al. 'Mindset interventions are a scalable treatment for academic underachievement' *Psychological Science* 26.6 (2015): 784–93.

5. Burnette, J. L. et al. 'Mind-sets matter: A meta-analytic review of implicit theories and self-regulation' *Psychological Bulletin* 139.3 (2013): 655–701.
6. Dweck, C. S. *Mindset: The new psychology of success* (Random House Publishing Group, 2006).
7. Blackwell, L. S. et al. 'Implicit theories of intelligence predict achievement across an adolescent transition: A longitudinal study and an intervention. *Child Development* 78.1 (2007): 246–63.
8. Ryan, R. M. & Deci, E. L. 'Self-determination theory and the facilitation of intrinsic motivation, social development, and well-being' *American Psychologist* 55.1 (2000): 68.
9. Yeager, D. S. & Dweck, C. S. 'Mindsets that promote resilience: When students believe that personal characteristics can be developed' *Educational Psychologist* 47.4 (2012): 302–14.

## Chapter 30: Love Yourself Slimmer: The Science of Self-Compassion

1. Neff, K. D. *Self-compassion: The proven power of being kind to yourself* (William Morrow, 2011).
2. Kristeller, J. L. & Quillian-Wolever, R. E. 'Mindfulness-based eating awareness training for treating binge eating disorder: The conceptual foundation' *Eating Disorders: The Journal of Treatment & Prevention* 19.1 (2011): 49–61.
3. Breines, J. G. & Chen, S. 'Self-compassion increases self-improvement motivation' *Personality and Social Psychology Bulletin* 38.9 (2012): 1133–43.
4. Cousineau, T. M. & Neff, K. D. 'Self-compassion and body dissatisfaction in women: A randomized controlled trial of a brief self-compassion intervention' *Mindfulness* 5.5 (2014): 444–54.
5. McGonigal, K. *The Willpower Instinct: How self-control works, why it matters, and what you can do to get more of it* (Avery, 2011).

## Chapter 31: Liberate Yourself With Healthy Eating

1. Lowe, M. R. et al. 'Dieting and restrained eating as prospective predictors of weight gain' *Frontiers in Psychology* 4 (2013): 577.
2. Conlin, H. J. et al. 'Flexible vs. rigid dieting in resistance-trained individuals seeking to optimize their physiques: A randomized controlled trial' *Journal of the International Society of Sports Nutrition* 18.1 (2021): 12.

3. Chin, S. H. & So, W. Y. 'The effects of weight fluctuation on the components of metabolic syndrome: A 16-year prospective cohort study in South Korea.' *Archives of Public Health* 79.1 (2021): 22.
4. Mann, T. et al. 'Medicare's search for effective obesity treatments: Diets are not the answer' *American Psychologist* 62.3 (2007): 220–33.
5. Lowe, M. R. et al. 'Dietary restraint and binge eating are associated with emotion regulation difficulties' *Appetite* 108 (2017): 40–4.
6. Tylka, T. L. et al. 'Intuitive eating and its impact on BMI and psychological health' *Journal of Obesity* (2015): 1–7.
7. Estruch, R. et al. 'Primary prevention of cardiovascular disease with a Mediterranean diet' *New England Journal of Medicine* 368.14 (2013): 1279–90.
8. Martinez-Gonzalez, M. A. et al. 'Benefits of the Mediterranean diet: Insights from the PREDIMED study' *BioMed Central Medicine* 12.1 (2014): 207.
9. Ahmad, S. et al. 'Assessment of risk factors and biomarkers associated with risk of cardiovascular disease among women consuming a Mediterranean diet' *Journal of the American Medical Association Network* 1.2 (2018): 1–13.

# About the Author

Sandra Roycroft-Davis DipCHyp, HPD, NLP Master Prac., MNCH is a visionary in the field of behavioural change, dedicated to helping people transform their lives. Her story isn't just about overcoming personal challenges; it's about sparking positive change in others around the world.

Sandra's early life was tough. Her mother often reminded her that the odds were against her, but Sandra held on to a firm belief in growth, positivity and kindness. Despite facing the harsh reality of being overweight, she made a promise to herself: her past wouldn't define her future. This commitment was the catalyst for her journey towards self-empowerment and change.

Determined to grow and stay kind, Sandra started a transformative journey. This path not only changed her own life but also inspired thousands of others. Through her dedication and training, she has become one of Britain's leading behavioural change specialists and has developed the Slimpod programme, a unique approach to weight loss that uses the power of the mind to transform people's relationship with food.

Sandra's story shows the strength of the human spirit and how one person can make a big difference. Today, she continues to inspire and guide others, promoting values like growth, positivity, kindness and responsibility. Her work helps people find their own paths to empowerment and lasting change.

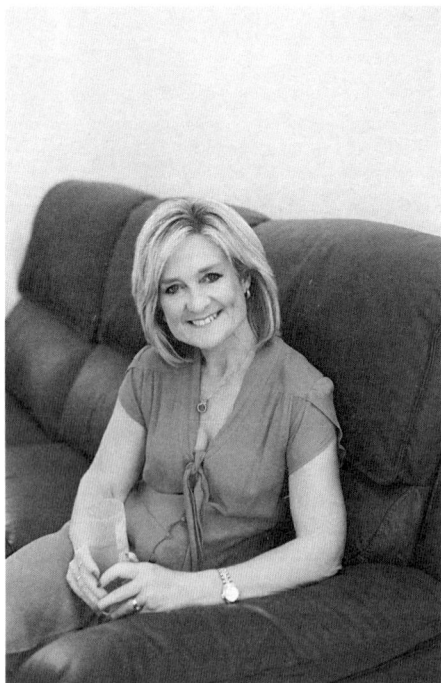

# Index

# INDEX